The Etherized Wife

The Etherized Wife

Privilege and Power in Sex Therapy Discourse

LESLIE MARGOLIN

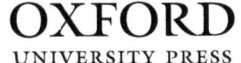

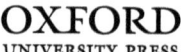

Oxford University Press is a department of the University of Oxford. It furthers
the University's objective of excellence in research, scholarship, and education
by publishing worldwide. Oxford is a registered trade mark of Oxford University
Press in the UK and certain other countries.

Published in the United States of America by Oxford University Press
198 Madison Avenue, New York, NY 10016, United States of America.

© Oxford University Press 2021

All rights reserved. No part of this publication may be reproduced, stored in
a retrieval system, or transmitted, in any form or by any means, without the
prior permission in writing of Oxford University Press, or as expressly permitted
by law, by license, or under terms agreed with the appropriate reproduction
rights organization. Inquiries concerning reproduction outside the scope of the
above should be sent to the Rights Department, Oxford University Press, at the
address above.

You must not circulate this work in any other form
and you must impose this same condition on any acquirer.

Library of Congress Cataloging-in-Publication Data
Names: Margolin, Leslie, 1945– author.
Title: The etherized wife : privilege and power in sex therapy discourse /
Leslie Margolin.
Description: New York : Oxford University Press, 2021. |
Includes bibliographical references and index.
Identifiers: LCCN 2020033755 (print) | LCCN 2020033756 (ebook) |
ISBN 9780190061203 (hardback) | ISBN 9780190061227 (epub) |
ISBN 9780190061234
Subjects: LCSH: Sex therapy. | Sex therapy—Case studies. |
Sex (Psychology)—Case studies. | Sex differences (Psychology)
Classification: LCC RC557 .M37 2021 (print) | LCC RC557 (ebook) |
DDC 616.85/8306—dc23
LC record available at https://lccn.loc.gov/2020033755
LC ebook record available at https://lccn.loc.gov/2020033756

DOI: 10.1093/oso/9780190061203.001.0001

What shimmers and bounces off the mirrored walls of the therapy room are reflections of dominant discourses that are as pervasive as the air we breathe.
   Rachel T. Hare-Mustin, "Discourses in the Mirrored Room"

A "political anatomy," which was also a "mechanics of power," was being born; it defined how one may have a hold over others' bodies, not only so that they may do what one wishes, but so that they may operate as one wishes, with the techniques, the speed and the efficiency that one determines. Thus discipline produces subjected and practiced bodies, "docile" bodies.
   Michel Foucault, *Discipline and Punish*

Contents

Introduction ... 1
    How the Research Began ... 8
    How the Book Is Organized ... 10

PART 1   SEX THERAPY PREHISTORY

1. Freud, Dora, and Compulsory Sexuality ... 21
    Dora's Story—An Overview ... 23
    Freud's Sexual Fixations ... 23
    Dora's Dreams ... 26
    A Masturbation Interrogation ... 28

2. The Frigidity Epidemic ... 32
    The New Definition ... 34
    A Master Lens ... 36
    Women Are to Blame ... 38
    Measuring Frigidity ... 41
    Constructing Normal Women ... 44

PART 2   BIRTH OF SEX THERAPY

3. Masters and Johnson and the Primacy of Intercourse ... 49
    Women's Liberation—On Men's Terms ... 51
    Intercourse *Ueber Alles* ... 55
    Freudians versus Masters and Johnson ... 64
    A Sensory Subject ... 67

4. Male Identification ... 73
    Helen Singer Kaplan ... 73
    The Myth of Equivalency ... 74
    Men's Sexual Sensitivity ... 76
    A Wife in Bondage ... 79
    Sexual Anorexia ... 81
    A Prisoner of Sex ... 85

5. Docile Bodies ... 88
    Systematic Desensitization ... 92
    The Intercourse Imperative ... 100
    When Sex Therapists Prescribe Intercourse ... 102

PART 3 CONTEMPORARY SEX THERAPY

6. Doublethink 109
   - Motivational Context Not Needed 110
   - The Language of Sensory Experience 112
   - Strategic Ignorance 114
   - Women's Sexual Desire Is Complicated 118
   - Prioritizing Sexual Coercion from an Earlier Time . . . 121

7. Men's Free Will 125
   - When a Man Feels Zero Desire 125
   - A Wife Must Adapt 126
   - Double-Consciousness 132
   - Masculine Exceptionalism 134

8. Women's Duty 137
   - She Takes One for the Team 138
   - Who Owns Mrs. D.'s Vagina? 142
   - Denying the Possibility of Sexual Coercion 143
   - Denying the Reality of Sexual Coercion 145

9. Sex Therapy Without Male Privilege and Power 148
   - A Focus on Inequality 148
   - A Focus on the Relationship 151
   - Externalizing the Problem 153

10. Discontinuities, Deviations, and Reversals 155
    - The Velvet Glove 156
    - Training Her Softly 160
    - Foregrounding the Relationship 161
    - Giving Women a Voice 163

Conclusion 167
   - How Does Sex Therapy Survive? 171
   - Can Sex Therapy Change? 173
   - Where Do We Go from Here? 175

Acknowledgments 179
Notes 181
Bibliography 205
Index 219

Introduction

> Not rape, not quite that, but undesired nevertheless, undesired to the core. As though she had decided to go slack, die within herself for the duration, like a rabbit when the jaws of the fox close on its neck. So that everything done to her might be done, as it were, far away.
> —J. M. Coetzee, *Disgrace* (1999)

In 1862, Dr. J. Marion Sims, an American surgeon specializing in women's diseases, opened a clinic in London where he heard a most unusual story. It was of a woman, married at the age of twenty-one, who could not copulate with her husband. The slightest touch at the entry to her vagina produced excruciating pain. After five or six weeks of painful and ineffectual exertion, the couple agreed to consult their family physician who conjectured that the failure was due to the smallness of the wife's genital organs, the largeness of the husband's, or both, and suggested that they try having intercourse while the wife is in a ether-induced coma. This was done and the intercourse accomplished without discomfort, but when the couple attempted intercourse the next day without ether, the discomfort returned. After a week of strenuous and fruitless effort, the family physician was sent for again, the wife was again etherized, and again copulation was effected without a hitch. However, as before, when they attempted intercourse without ether, the pain was unbearable.[1]

The family physician described the husband as "tall, athletic, and muscular... not subject to hasty ejaculation," in possession of "extraordinary copulative powers," which led him to believe that the problem led back, entirely, to the wife.[2] The only remedy he could offer was to etherize her whenever the need to copulate arose. Suffice it to say that the physician soon began visiting this couple's residence two or three times a week to etherize the woman for the purpose of easing copulation. They persevered in this manner for a whole year, when conception occurred. During the gestation period, they continued to use etherization to facilitate coition, but hoped that after the child's birth, it would not be necessary. But that was not to be the case. After the birth, the couple managed to copulate a few times without ether, but each copulation was so painful that they felt they had no choice but to return to ether again. After another year of ethereal copulation, there was a second pregnancy that ended in miscarriage. Yet another year passed with constant etherization, when at last they became alarmed at their dependency on ether and the coma it produced and decided to give it up altogether.

Three or four more years passed without copulation, nor any effort at copulation, when the couple consulted with Dr. Sims. Examination of the wife's genitalia revealed excessive sensitivity of the hymen and vulvar outlet, coupled with an involuntary spasmodic contraction of the vaginal sphincter muscle at the least contact, in other words, vaginismus, a disease that Sims is credited with discovering and naming. In this instance, notwithstanding the fact that the patient had accomplished coition scores, perhaps hundreds of times, and that a full-term birth had also occurred, the spasmodic contractions of the vaginal sphincter were so intense that Dr. Sims could barely insert his index finger.

In an effort to nullify the contractions and make her vagina more accommodating, Dr. Sims placed the fully etherized wife on her back and with his scalpel removed the whole ring of tissue that encircled the mouth of her vagina. He then divided the septum between the fourchette and rectum on both sides, "down through the fibers of the sphincter muscle and the fourchette to the perineal raphe," leaving an extremely narrow partition between the two outlets. Then a glass dilator was introduced into her vagina and worn almost constantly, until it was replaced in a day or two by a larger dilator. In two weeks, sexual intercourse was accomplished for the first time without pain.[3]

Unlike cliteridectomy and ovariotomy (the surgical removal of the clitoris and ovaries as treatments for masturbation and a host of other moral and psychological disorders[4]), vaginismus surgery inspired no inflated rhetoric either in support or condemnation. Even at the very moment Dr. Sims invented the surgery, it gave rise to little praise, except, perhaps, from Sims himself, who declared his surgical cure an unmitigated success: "From personal observation I can confidently assert that I know of no disease capable of producing so much unhappiness to both parties of the marriage contract, and I am happy to state that I know of no serious trouble that can be cured so easily, so safely, and so certainly."[5] In 1887, Dr. T. Moore Madden, echoing the position of the British medical community, registered full agreement with the first part of Sim's assessment, but with regard to the second half, Sim's reference to the easy curability of the disease via surgery, he regretted that his own experience was by no means as satisfactory. For while he believed that surgical procedures directed to curing the contractions and pain of vaginismus, such as the excision of the hymen and deep incisions into the vagina, may have a place in certain cases of vaginismus, in quite as many cases they are unnecessary: "[F]rom my own clinical experience I can vouch for the possibility in some cases of relieving the most intense dyspareunia resulting from this cause, so as to enable the patient to fulfill all her duties as a wife and eventually as a mother, without any operation beyond the forcible mechanical expansion of the vaginal canal."[6]

By the beginning of the twentieth century, surgery, as the premier treatment of vaginismus, was dying out, though from time to time, it flickered briefly back to life.[7] The main process at work in this slow obsolescence was the growing conviction that a woman's resistance to intercourse, as characterized by the spasmodic contractions of her vagina, is psychological in origin. The one most responsible for this shift is Freud. After Freud, the question was no longer simply, "Is there something about the woman's vagina that may be blocking intercourse?" but also "What does intercourse mean to her?" "What part of her history does intercourse recall?" "What does she gain, or imagine herself gaining, by blocking intercourse?" It was no longer simply: "At what point does the mouth of her vagina go into spasms?" but "How can we translate her spasms into language?" "What message is her vagina trying to communicate by reacting in this way?" It was no longer simply "How can we change the structure of her vagina?" but "What kind of insight or emotional cleansing (abreaction) would be most helpful?" "How can we change her understanding of intercourse?"

Of course, these generalizations require some qualification. To begin with, Freud's influence on sex therapy did not materialize all at once or as part of a single process. More than forty years elapsed before Freud's belief "that sexuality is the key to the problem of the psychoneuroses and of the neuroses in general"[8] evolved into the idea that vaginismus is not a disease, in itself, but a symptom of an underlying neurosis held in place by a complex network of unconscious forces, as Otto Fenichel would one day clarify in his *Psychoanalytic Theory of Neurosis*: "Vaginismus is related to frigidity as reaction formation is to repression; not only is the sexual excitement inhibited, but something positive is done to ensure the maintenance of such an inhibition and to make intercourse physically impossible . . . ; it then not only expresses the tendency to offer an obstacle to sexuality but also a distorted unconscious wish."[9]

After Freud, psychiatric discourses on sexuality became expansive, diffuse, and elusive, and as a consequence, the treatments that once depended on a scalpel and scissors came to depend on a variety of new techniques directed to thoughts, feelings, and behaviors, many of which embraced the goal of changing not only how a woman copulated, but how she understood copulation, what she wanted from it, feared about it, and how she came to see it in those ways. Some of these techniques may have been less concerned with understanding than with extinguishing dysfunctional symptoms as rapidly as possible, but the dark side, what they all retained as their singular purpose, is the control of a woman's sexuality, the accomplishment of which depended on treating her sexual functions as the central and most valid representation of her personality. As a result of this focus, an entire corpus of knowledge, theory, and techniques—"systems of micropower that are essentially non-egalitarian and asymmetrical"[10]—developed around the question of how to take a woman's sexuality for the whole of her and, in so doing, how to turn her into a better (and more cooperative) sexual performer.

This book is intended as a genealogy of these discourses, in particular, a genealogy of how psychiatrists, psychologists, social workers, sexologists, and counselors came to advocate heterosexual intercourse without overtly acknowledging or recognizing the effects of that advocacy: the legitimation of male sexuality and male supremacy. To say this another way, this book is about how the etherized wife is still with us, and for the same reasons.[11] The general argument may be called *gender imperialism*. It holds that in sex, like other domains of life in which men set the standard of normality, women have been judged normal to the degree they match men's expectations.[12] This book seeks to examine, in historical perspective, how this judgment has been articulated and supported by the discipline responsible for treating women's sexual problems—sex therapy.

A second, and equally central goal for this research, is to move outside the space of conventional sex therapy discourse to focus upon and learn how sex therapy, as a discipline, has been constituted by a series of assumptions and sustained through practices which treat those assumptions as true. I examine how these foundational assumptions, which comprise what I shall call the *intercourse imperative*,[13] are so deeply taken for granted, and applied so subtly in sex therapy practice, that therapists, in their therapeutic and academic discourses, not only fail to question them; they often fail to acknowledge their existence.

One of these assumptions is that penis–vagina intercourse is natural, necessary, and healthful, a phenomenon beyond critical analysis, an assumption shared by America, and by Western society, as a whole.[14] As Andrea Dworkin put it,

> In Amerika, there is the nearly universal conviction—or so it appears—that sex (fucking) is good and that liking it is right: morally right; a sign of human health; nearly a standard for citizenship.[15]

This implies a second assumption, which is that those who abstain from intercourse, either because they lack interest, find sex aversive, or because they cannot become aroused, are either physically or mentally ill, hence the proliferation of medical/psychiatric diagnoses such as "inhibited sexual desire disorder," "aversive sexual desire disorder," "hypoactive sexual desire disorder," and "female sexual interest/arousal disorder."

A third, related assumption is that everyone is sexual, whether they know it or not, and that their sexuality influences virtually every human activity. As one sex therapist wrote:

If we observe people carefully, virtually every action one witnesses will have some connection to sexuality. . . . It organizes identities, the way we perceive others, and the way others judge us. It guides our vocational efforts and our quest for status and recognition. Sexuality guides our speech, our gestures, the way we walk, our willingness to fight or flee, and even our assessment of beauty.[16]

A fourth assumption is that women in long-term relationships with men engage in sexual intercourse of their own free will. This assumption derives from the social convention that once a woman has intercourse with a man, her consent for all future sexual activity with him is effectively taken for granted.[17]

A fifth assumption is that, while oral and manual activity can pass as sex, "actual" or "real" sex for heterosexual couples consists of penis–vagina penetration, followed by the penis thrusting inside the vagina, and ending in orgasms for both partners.[18] To put this somewhat differently, sex therapists' definition of "the act" has tended to correspond with most laypeople's definition, and also with what we see in pornography and in popular media, a definition consistent with the status quo of male dominance and female subordination.[19]

This implies a final assumption, which is that a woman has both the capacity and obligation to coordinate her sexual needs and responses to those of her male partner, but that no reciprocal obligation exists for her male partner to coordinate his sexual needs and responses to hers. The underlying message: it is unnecessary to consider women's anatomic, psychological, and socioeconomic differences, unnecessary to consider that women "do not express or report or exhibit as much interest in having sex as men do,"[20] and, furthermore, unnecessary to consider evidence such as a recent national probability sample of women's sexual desire, which found that as many as 26.7% of premenopausal women and 52.4% of menopausal women report little interest in intercourse.[21]

Intercourse should work fine for women. And when it doesn't, women should be sanctioned and corrected for their failure. As Toni Morrison showed in *The Bluest Eye*, when a disempowered group cannot live up to the standards of the empowered group due to their physiological differences, the disempowered will still be judged by the standards of the empowered.[22] To cite Rachel Hare-Mustin and Jeanne Maracek's *Making a Difference: Psychology and the Construction of Gender* (1990), "As long as male behavior remains the standard in the culture, women's differences from men will be regarded as deficiencies."[23] Thus, when one heterosexual man, a participant in a study on intercourse, was asked how he would respond to a sexual partner who preferred to do something other than intercourse, he could barely contain his disappointment and astonishment:

Hm. I might, um I dunno. I could find it, I mean it could be viewed as being selfish but um I, yeah. I think I, I would, well I'd start to ask "why?" "Why, why, what is like wrong with me and wrong with you, and this [is] what I see as perfectly normal behaviour. Um why is it wrong for you?"[24]

Intercourse works for men; it is what they want, and it almost always brings them to orgasm. Unfortunately, if we are to believe social science research, intercourse, in the majority of cases, is far less successful for women.[25] According to one study, over ninety percent of women reach orgasm easily via clitoral massage or masturbation, but only two percent actually insert something into their vagina while they stimulate themselves to orgasm.[26] As early as the 1950s, Kinsey found that masturbation focused on the clitoris is how "the female most frequently reaches orgasm."[27] The message could not be any clearer. The clitoris, and not the interior of the vagina, is the center of sexual stimulation and sensation for women. That women do not mimic the thrusting motions of a penis when attempting to bring themselves to orgasm points to a mismatch between the type of stimulation that women are expected to have (and want) during sex with a man and the type of stimulation that works best for them. One consequence of this mismatch, quite apart from the fact that it leaves women sexually dissatisfied,[28] is that it often makes women feel as though there is something wrong with them. They often feel that, because they cannot respond to intercourse in the prescribed way, at the prescribed moment, they are abnormal, unhealthy, deficient. In this book, I argue that this is one of the most notable, and ironic, achievements of the intercourse imperative: to hold women accountable for transgressing rules established by men for their own advantage and to get those who are involved, women as well as men, to agree that it is women who are behaving inappropriately in sexual situations in which they are dominated. The growing literature on women's subjective experience during intercourse is filled with evidence of this kind of asymmetric judgment—confessions of women's self-reproach and self-doubt. As one woman described her feelings,

> I think that a lot of my desire to have orgasms during intercourse comes from shame and feelings of inadequacy (maybe I'm not sexy...). Hell, I don't know—I've been in therapy for two years and it has helped me personally, but I'm still no closer to having an orgasm during intercourse.[29]

The failure to feel aroused or have orgasms during intercourse not only makes women feel as though they are not "real" or "normal" women, but their male partner's conviction that they should experience orgasm from his continued thrusting often makes him feel disappointed and insecure, either by making him wonder about his performance ("What am I doing wrong?") or by making him wonder about his partner's sexuality ("What's wrong with her?"). As a consequence of this failure to live up to the male standard of sexuality, women have been subject to judgment and condemnation. Because women in general are less interested in intercourse than men, less easily aroused by intercourse, and less likely to experience orgasm from it,[30] they are more likely to receive psychiatric diagnoses. They are more likely to be seen as mentally ill.

This book examines sex therapy's role in this inequity. It considers the possibility that, under the assumption that sex therapists are helping heterosexual women enjoy healthier, happier, and more fulfilling sexual intercourse—under the assumption that they are giving heterosexual women what they want and need—they have inadvertently pushed women to adapt to a male model of sexuality. Which is not to say women have not wanted intercourse to work for themselves and their partners. They have.[31] It is to say, rather, that many of the reasons women want intercourse to work may have been misinterpreted, ignored, or devalued in sex therapy—specifically, the reasons that have little to do with physiological sensation and orgasm, and everything to do with accommodation and even survival. As Andrea Dworkin interpreted women's sexual motivations,

> [w]e are poorer than men in money and so we have to barter sex or sell it outright (which is why they keep us poorer in money). We are poorer than men in psychological well-being because for us self-esteem depends on the approval—frequently expressed through sexual desire—of those who have and exercise power over us.... We need their money; intercourse is frequently how we get it. We need their approval to be able to survive inside our own skins; intercourse is frequently how we get it.[32]

When men's and women's social and economic inequality are ignored as a condition of their sexual interaction, it is easy to lose sight of the possibility that women have been performing under duress. When we strip heterosexual relationships of socio-economic context, we may not notice when a woman's sexual survival involves a performance strategy known as "passing" in which she presents herself as more interested in intercourse (and sex therapy) than she really is to avoid disapproval and the appearance abnormality.[33] She may communicate misleading information based on her internalization of social scripts that demand the performance of friendliness, deference, compliance, and the affirmation and celebration of men's achievements,[34] a phenomenon that explains a variety of common, gender specific symptoms such as faking sexual arousal and orgasm,[35] tolerating or suppressing sexual pain,[36] and prioritizing a partner's pleasure over her own.[37]

This investigation examines the possibility that sex therapy has inadvertently represented intercourse as the "natural" way for women to have sex and experience orgasm. For example, when Joseph Wolpe, the behavioral psychologist, described his "impotent" patient's intercourse experience with this sentence, "He ejaculated prematurely on the first occasion but later performed very successfully," he was not advocating for the rightness and necessity of intercourse for women.[38] He did not even refer to women's orgasm or sexual pleasure. His meaning was simply understood, too obvious to require an explanation: a man is impotent, a failure at intercourse, when he cannot delay ejaculation long enough to bring his female partner to orgasm, and he is successful when he can.[39]

This investigation reveals that sex therapy often treats this definition of sexual success as self-evident. For heterosexual men to perform intercourse correctly, they need to continue thrusting long enough to bring a woman to orgasm.[40] This is the measure of men's sexual success. Yet sex therapy has not provided a justification for this measure, nor has it acknowledged the need for such a justification. Following Thomas Kuhn, *The Etherized Wife* presents a view of "normal" sex therapy as a puzzle-solving activity in which the "paradigm" that organizes sex therapy knowledge—the intercourse imperative—is treated, not as a hypothesis that therapists or scholars test against reality, but as the reality from which sex therapy proceeds.[41]

How the Research Began

To support these claims, I map a series of case studies illustrating sex therapy's central approaches to heterosexual couples and, also, to a lesser degree, sex therapy's approaches to lesbian couples. However, before I begin, for the sake of transparency, it might be helpful to explain how I adopted a case-study methodology and how I decided to highlight certain therapists and case studies.

About five or six years ago, as I was engaged in a research project about mid-twentieth century psychiatry, I came upon an article in a 1969 issue of the *British Journal of Psychiatry*[42] that described how a behavioral sex therapist—the article's author—encouraged the husband of his patient to penetrate her vagina despite her objections: to force his way in. (I discuss this case study at the close of chapter 5, "Docile Bodies.") This inspired me to begin exploring the sex therapy literature, from as early as the Victorian era through the present day, to see if there were more cases like this. I found that there were. In going through the textbooks, journal articles, and case-study collections, I found no cases in which a sex therapist supported a woman's right to abstain from sex, despite her objections, when her partner was a man. This surprised me, even though other sex therapy scholars—led by Leonore Tiefer[43]—had already taken note of sex therapy's pro-male bias. What surprised me even more is that, after checking how these studies were cited, I noted that the academics who cited them, cited them as examples of how sex therapy should be conducted. Moreover, these citations were not limited to the decade or era when the article was published. For instance, the 1969 article by the psychiatrist who encouraged the husband of his female patient to force intercourse was cited six times during the 1990s and six times more in the current millennium. And the citations were always positive. This led me to conclude that sexism in sex therapy is not a matter of this or that therapist's pro-male bias; it's a systemic problem, and it's a problem that continues to this day. I also concluded that the best way to understand this continuity is to begin with sex therapy's originators and that the best way to see how sex therapy may have favored men's interests over women's is to focus on cases where partners present fundamental differences in sexual desire, where one partner wants more sex and the other less, a problem that has long been the main reason women seek, are referred to, or are pressured to attend sex therapy.[44] The guiding principle of case selection, then, was not to establish whether sexism exists among sex therapists, nor was I looking for the most egregious or most cited case studies. Rather, my goal was to examine how this gender bias originated, how it works, how it might be maintained, and why it goes unnoticed. Thus, I selected cases that offered the clearest examples of the multiple ways sex therapists transmit and reinforce the male-serving assumption that intercourse is the desirable, natural outcome of sex therapy.

I would also like to share a second reason for undertaking this research. As someone who trained at a Freudian psychoanalytic institute during the 1970s, I was, for quite some time, a passionate follower of Freud. However, as the years passed, and as I became more involved in my academic career, that passion largely dissolved, except, that is, for one core Freudian tenet: the notion that everyone is inherently sexual, the notion that everyone, whether they know it or not, is driven by sexual desire. My belief in that tenet only began to erode recently as a result of something that began happening in my Human Sexuality classes. At about the same time I discovered the article about the psychiatrist who encouraged forced intercourse, more and more of my students—primarily women—began coming out to the class as asexual.[45] My relationships with them prompted me to begin studying asexuality and prompted me, further, to begin thinking about how psychiatrists and other types of professionals engaged in sex therapy have, for decades, regarded the absence of sexual desire as abnormal—as pathology. Thus, my case study investigation began to focus on how the Freudian belief in the universality and preeminence of sexual desire influenced sex therapy—in particular, how that core belief interacted with gender norms, placing women at a disadvantage.

My study of gender bias in sex therapy, then, is drawn from the texts—handbooks, collections, articles, and demonstration videos—that have been, and continue to be, treated as exemplars of the field's collective consciousness. I focus, in other words, on studies written by and for professional sex therapists on how to conduct successful sex therapy. For the contemporary period, for example, I focus on texts such as the *Handbook of Clinical Sexuality for Mental Health Professionals, Principles and Practice of Sex Therapy, The Wiley Handbook of Sex Therapy, Systemic Sex Therapy, Handbook of Sexual Dysfunction, Case Studies in Sex Therapy, Quickies: The Handbook of Brief Sex Therapy, DSM Casebooks, DSM Clinical Cases, Casebook for DSM-5*, and peer-reviewed periodicals such as the *Journal of Marital and Family Therapy, Journal of Family Psychotherapy, Journal of Sex & Marital Therapy, The Family Journal, American Journal of Family Therapy, Sexual and Relationship Therapy*, and *Journal of Homosexuality*. While the case studies contained in these texts are always incomplete in the sense that they never provide the totality of what the therapist and patient said—they should never be taken as a literal recording of events—they do represent therapists' and authors' priorities. They represent what therapists and authors want us to know.

I chose to focus on some case studies over others for two main reasons: for their prominence in the history of sex therapy (thus my concentration on Freud, Masters and Johnson, Kaplan, Wolpe, and Hartman and Fithian), and for their relevance to what Foucault called "the various systems of subjugation" and "the endlessly repeated play of dominations."[46] Most of the case studies selected for inclusion, then, represent a kind of treatment that seems unfair and oppressive to women, a kind of treatment, specifically, where women's right to say "no" to intercourse goes unrecognized or unappreciated. In line with this, while I found several case studies that support a man's right to abstain from sex with his female partner and others that affirm a woman's right to abstain from sex with her female partner, I did not find any that support a woman's right to abstain from sex with her male partner. This book's goal is to better understand this gender difference, both in terms of its underlying logic and how it influences sex therapy practice.

How the Book Is Organized

Foucault does not elaborate, in any direct way, what he means by a genealogical history,[47] but he does offer some relatively clear examples in *Discipline and Punish* and *The History of Sexuality, Vol. 1*, where he shows how historical data should be used to perform a genealogical analysis. As he writes in *Discipline and Punish*:

> I would like to write a history of this prison, with all the political investments of the body that it gathers together in its closed architecture. Why? Simply because

I am interested in the past? No, if one means by that writing a history of the past in terms of the present. Yes, if one means writing a history of the present.[48]

To restate Foucault's position, a genealogy is less concerned with understanding the past, than it is with using historical materials to critically reframe the present. And that is what I hope to accomplish here. My interest in a genealogical approach to sex therapy arises from my discovery of an unexplored, unacknowledged continuity between sex therapy from earlier times and contemporary practice. And like Foucault, I am interested in systems of constraint and subjugation. As Foucault told an interviewer in 1971, "My problem is essentially the definition of the implicit systems in which we find ourselves prisoners: what I would like to grasp is the system of limits and exclusion which we practice without knowing it; I would like to make the cultural unconscious apparent."[49]

While the book is divided into three historical sections, Prehistory of Sex Therapy, Birth of Sex Therapy, and Contemporary Sex Therapy, for the most part, I did not adhere to any rigid time frames. For the Prehistory and Birth sections, for example, I was mainly concerned with including the most influential and typical therapists, techniques, and authors. Thus, the Prehistory section begins with Freud's demonstration of how to impose male sexuality onto a patient he renamed "Dora."[50] While Dora, an adolescent girl, did not seek him out to receive help for a sexual discrepancy issue, I show that a sexual discrepancy did surface during her treatment, the discrepancy between the way Dora's male therapist interpreted her sexuality and the way she interpreted her own. Although the "talking cure" Freud imposed on Dora may not have been physically painful or injurious, it was similar in its basic assumptions to the ethereal and surgical cures it replaced. Freud erased Dora as a knowing person.[51] He forced Dora to affirm sexual identities, desires, and behaviors that were not her own; he insisted, despite her vigorous denials and the absence of confirmatory evidence, that she was always driven by sexual motivation. As the chapters in the Birth of Sex Therapy and Contemporary Sex Therapy sections will show, Freud's belief in the omnipresence and power of sexual desire—his belief in the undeniability of sexual desire—forms one of the dominant narratives of the sex therapy discipline.

In the chapter that follows, I examine how the next generation of Freudian therapists, by invoking sexual "frigidity" theory, cast women who did not live up to men's sexual expectations as psychosocial deviants requiring the strictest oversight and management, a category of people who, like Dora, deserve little credibility as tellers of their own sexual stories.[52] While this chapter focuses on the hostility therapists directed toward women, the condemnation and silencing of those who rejected their husbands' sexual overtures, I also show how sexual frigidity discourse had a flipside: therapists valorized women who conformed to traditional feminine roles (as wife, mother, housekeeper, and compliant, attentive sex partner), holding them up as the gold standard of feminine normality.

The second third of the book is devoted to the launching of the sex therapy discipline—chronicling how, during the 1960s and 1970s, a group of therapists led by Masters and Johnson, Helen Singer Kaplan, Joseph Wolpe, and Hartman and Fithian, adapted a series of new, short-term, behavioral approaches to the treatment of people's sex problems. These therapists differed from their Freudian counterparts in their emphasis on scientific research and education, on changing patients' negative, puritanical sexual attitudes to positive liberated attitudes, and their practice of prescribing sexual exercises and techniques. At the same time, behaviorally oriented therapists implicitly maintained the Freudian tenets: everyone is motivated by an inborn, omnipresent fount of sexual desire; intercourse is the healthiest, most natural way to express that desire; and men's sexual needs trump women's.

The final third of the book focuses on contemporary sex therapy. I chose 1980 as the beginning of the contemporary period because that was the year that the *Diagnostic and Statistical Manual of Mental Disorders* (*DSM-III*) shifted from a clinically based psychoanalytic model to a research-based medical model.[53] According to the task force charged with designing this new model, a psychiatric disorder had to demonstrate two essential features: subjective distress and a general impairment in social or mental functioning.[54] As a result, the *DSM-III* conceptualized a psychiatric disorder as "a clinically significant behavioral or psychological syndrome or pattern that occurs in an individual that is typically associated with either a painful symptom (distress) or impairment in one or more areas of functioning."[55] Members of the *DSM-III* task force also concluded that a behavioral or psychological syndrome or pattern had to be *inherently* distressful or maladaptive and not distressful and maladaptive due to conflict between the psychological pattern and a specific environment. As members of the task force explained, "If the negative consequences occur in all environments, the condition is a disorder. If they occur in special environments, then the condition is considered a vulnerability."[56] Ironically, the *DSM-III*, the first *Diagnostic and Statistical Manual* specifically oriented to a research-based medical model, was also the first to list "inhibited sexual desire" as a psychiatric disorder, despite the absence of research suggesting that having little or no interest in sex is associated with distress and impaired functioning.

This section of the book reveals that following publication of the *DSM-III*, sex therapy disadvantaged women in much the same ways they had been disadvantaged in earlier eras. As before, psychiatrists and other sex therapists skipped over the question of how power is divided and expressed in a woman's heterosexual relationship; for decades after the *DSM-III* was published, the social/

relational context affecting a woman's putative sexual dysfunction was treated as irrelevant. What mattered, only, was how sexually responsive she was.

Eventually the American Psychiatric Association came to recognize that eliding the social/relationship context in which a woman's alleged sexual dysfunction occurs had been a mistake. The first move in the direction of acknowledging that mistake occurred in the *DSM-IV* (1994) where the American Psychiatric Association cautioned psychiatrists against diagnosing anyone with "low sexual desire" without first taking into account that "apparent 'low desire' in one partner may instead reflect an excessive need for sexual expression in the other partner."[57] Nineteen years later, the *DSM-5* (2013) took a more forceful position, amounting to a complete reversal, stipulating that "if interpersonal or significant cultural factors, such as severe relationship distress, intimate partner violence, or other significant stressors explain sexual interest/arousal symptoms, then a diagnosis of sexual interest/arousal disorder would not be made."[58] Both the *DSM-IV* and *DSM-5* provisos were late in coming out, and unfortunately, as the closing chapters reveal, they weren't followed very carefully, if at all. This might be partly because the *DSM-5* mentions only one kind of relationship stressor—"intimate partner violence"—but fails to specify other, much more common, relationship stressors such an nonviolent sexual coercion. A woman's male partner may react to her sexual performance with disappointment, anger, threats, and even verbal abuse, but these contingencies have not been sufficiently studied in the sex therapy literature. That's what I hope to clarify in this book; that's the gap my book attempts to fill. Among long-term heterosexual couples, nonviolent sexual coercion happens around intercourse, and happens often, and it makes a certain amount of sense that it would, given men's greater power and greater investment in intercourse.

The first chapter in this section, "Doublethink," explores seemingly contradictory standards in sex therapy that appear to deny, divert, and dismiss information suggesting that a woman's disinterest in sex may be a normal behavior variant or that it may be situationally specific—a reaction to her male partner's behavior. The next chapter, "Men's Free Will" examines how differently sex therapy can unfold when a heterosexual male presents with the problem of low sexual desire—how heterosexual men are often treated more respectfully, more attentively, and more generously than heterosexual women. The chapter that follows, "Women's Duty," mirrors the previous one, showing how intercourse has been treated as a husband's right and a wife's obligation. The penultimate chapter in this section, "Sex Therapy without Male Privilege and Power," examines what sex therapy looks like when the patients are lesbians. The final chapter, "Discontinuities, Deviations, and Reversals," illustrates how contemporary sex therapy discourse, while sharing several common features, often defies simple, one-dimensional characterizations.

The discussion of sex therapy with lesbian couples shows how sex therapy can recognize the socio-economic contexts of patients' lives and can achieve real, unbiased compromise between partners when they show a discrepancy in sexual interest. The lessons to be learned from sex therapy with women partnered with women are powerful, yet astonishingly simple (see the book's conclusion for a discussion of these lessons), but sexism is also powerful, with an incredible capacity to adapt and deceive. Consider, for example, this observation from Helen Singer Kaplan: "A healthy person cannot develop a gratifying marriage with someone who consistently and chronically frustrates him sexually despite his best efforts."[59] On the surface, there is nothing androcentric or misogynistic here. Kaplan is not saying anything specific about women or men. At the same time, since women are far more likely to lose interest in sex than men[60]—since they are the ones far more likely to say, "It would be okay with me if we never have sex again!"—Kaplan's observation has an implicit gender bias and can be used as a justification for extortion. She appears to be saying that only a weak or neurotic man would put up with a woman who withholds in this way and, thus, appears to be arguing in favor of a moral code that allows a man to threaten to leave a wife who frustrates him sexually.[61]

Under these circumstances, a wife who wants to keep her marriage may have very few sexual choices—in fact, the whole concept of sexual "choice" becomes controversial—as this *Dear Abby* letter illustrates:

> Dear Abby: Is it normal for men to sulk or get angry when they don't get sex when they want it? I've been married to my husband for more than 30 years. I run several miles a day and, with all the work I do, I don't always feel like having sex. Lately, I have been under a lot of stress, so I haven't been in the mood.
>
> The other night, he did his usual sulking. Then, as he often does, he tossed about in bed, repeatedly and roughly, while we're trying to sleep. The whole bed shook. Another night, he stuck his elbow in my ribs to be sure he got my attention.
>
> Sometimes he'll grab my butt really hard while I'm trying to sleep—in the middle of the night, mind you. I end up having sex with him so he leaves me alone and I can sleep.
>
> I have tried sleeping in another bed. But then he comes to that room and repeatedly kicks the mattress. If I lock the door, he kicks the door. So, I have sex with him so I can live in peace. Do most men do this when they don't get sex as often as they like?
>
> —*Spouse Sulking in The North* (August 9, 2017)

One of my main motivations for writing this book is the conviction that this *Dear Abby* letter represents the experience of many women and couples and that there is scant evidence that sex therapists are aware of it. Scant evidence that sex therapists are aware of the despair of women who resign themselves to intercourse because resistance is futile or dangerous or otherwise unimaginable. Scant evidence that they are aware that many of their women patients "consent" to intercourse, not because they welcome the experience—not because they are interested in orgasm or sensory stimulation—but because they perceive the consequences of resistance as more costly than the consequences of acquiescence.[62]

We know that in the 1950s and early 1960s, a sex therapist could unhesitatingly recommend that a wife with little interest in sex should work harder to meet her husband's sexual needs. ("When the wife behaves in bed as she thinks the 'other woman' would behave she is less likely to lose her husband. It is one of her duties not only to learn something about preparing meals, but she also should learn how to *satisfy her husband sexually* which in turn will result in her own greater happiness" [Caprio, *The Sexually Adequate Female*][63]). At mid-century, sex therapists routinely cautioned women against ever turning their man away. ("As a rule of thumb, I usually tell women *always* to meet their husbands' sexual requirements unless frank disability keeps them from performing their usual household or working duties or specific disorders of the sexual organs themselves make intercourse impossible" [Eichenlaub, *The Marriage Art*][64]). During this era, a sex therapist could openly recommend that wives pretend that they are enjoying intercourse and having orgasms, the better to satisfy their husbands' need to feel sexually skillful and potent. ("This is a great deal better than nothing for both partners and it frequently makes for a happy marriage. It is an instinctive expression of love and acceptance of responsibility in love on the wife's part and it gives her husband the confidence and pride in his male vigor that he needs—so long as he never suspects the deception" [Davis, *The Sexually Responsible* Woman][65]).

After second wave feminism, however, a sex therapist could not say anything remotely like this. A sex therapist who did would be seen as absurdly dated and inappropriate—anti-feminist and androcentric to the extreme. While this research suggests that sex therapists are no longer overtly biased in favor of men, that on the surface they fervently advocate for gender equality and female empowerment, it reveals that sex therapists' descriptions of their patients and the treatments they provide, as presented in their case studies, contain linkages to the discipline's sexist origins.

The canniest dimension of this sexism is that it is safely tucked away from view. It is so deeply engrained in sex therapy that, save for a few very special therapists, it remains unacknowledged, entirely outside everyday discourse. In the new era of data-driven, evidence-based practice, where "sex therapy focuses on proper technique and communication, with interventions assumed to be scientific, professional, objective, and value free,"[66] where there no longer seems to be a need to politicize professional services, therapists continue to behave as if the sexual activity most favored by men—intercourse—should be privileged over the sexual activities favored by women.[67] They continue to behave as if sexuality is an individual faculty or property, rather than something created in and through social interaction, and they continue to behave as if a woman's sexual problem is something akin to a bodily illness ("She seems to be suffering from female orgasmic disorder"), rather than something determined by her political, economic, and social inequality.[68] If sex therapists still behave in these ways, despite all that feminists have had to say about sexual inequality and inequity, then it is important to see how they carry these values into the therapy room and into therapeutic discourse. It is important to see how sex therapy, despite all the scientific research, continues to be a deeply political matter.

It goes without saying that many others have examined these issues before me. Rachel Hare-Mustin, Peggy Kleinplatz, Margaret Jackson, Jeanne Shaw, and Leonore Tiefer have provided a number of essential background and reference points, specifically, that sex therapy has been too focused on genitals; too goal oriented; too reliant on sexist research, language, and theory; too supportive of patriarchal interests normative sexual performance, and compulsory heterosexuality; and too uninterested in gender inequality, power differentials, and social causes. As Peggy Kleinplatz described contemporary sex therapy,

> [t]he values conveyed by the current model include maintaining the status quo, particularly a patriarchal sexual norm. There is an emphasis on objective, behavioral criteria—that is, sexual intercourse—as the ultimate end of sexual relations. There is little mention of self-expression, pleasure, or subjective satisfaction."[69]

I owe a special debt to Jeanne Shaw who anticipated the concept of the etherized wife more than twenty years before I began this investigation:

> The usual treatment of primary vaginismus consists essentially of shaping a woman's behavior to fit her partner's (and society's) expectation that she perform. Current treatment enables her to tolerate penetration, please her partner, and feel like a woman. These achievements help her feel functional and competent. Feeling functional, she now behaves on behalf of her partner to express herself through sexual intercourse.[70]

I am also indebted to Michel Foucault whose study of disciplinary power provided a model for this research, especially his argument that sexuality, like other forms of human experience, is rooted in discourse: constituted by "all the statements that named it, divided it up, described it, explained it, traced its development, indicated its correlations, judged it, and possibly gave it speech by articulating in its name, discourses that were to be taken as its own."[71] From this perspective, the power that sex therapists exercise over patients may appear "soft" in character, an example of what Miranda Fricker calls "identity power," for it operates by sharing conceptions of normal, healthy sex for men and women, gays and straights, young and old.[72] At the same time, following Marilyn Frye's lead, I argue that this kind of power can be just as oppressive as physical coercion. If sex therapy reflects men's interests and values, indeed, if it consistently devalues women's sexual needs and autonomy when they are seeking help with their long-term heterosexual relationships, it would, unknowingly, commit a fundamental kind of harm. As Frye explained, and as we will consider in the chapters which follow, it would commit *mayhem*: "a maiming which impairs a person's ability to defend herself. Mayhem is very close kin both morally and logically to murder."[73]

Finally, Andrea Dworkin's (1987) great work, *Intercourse*, inspired the basic idea driving this book, that what appears as consensual heterosexual intercourse—what appears as bloodless, painless, and absolutely normal—can also be understood as a tool of social domination,

> a form of possession or an act of possession in which, during which, because of which, a man inhabits a woman, physically covering her and overwhelming her and at the same time penetrating her; and this physical relation to her—over her and inside her—is his possession of her. He has her, or, when he is done, he has had her. By thrusting into her, he takes her over.... The sexual act that by its nature makes her his.[74]

To those who read Dworkin's words as wildly eccentric, the point of view of a bitter, man-hating fanatic, consider how Theodor Van de Velde described intercourse in much the same way in his *Ideal Marriage* (1926), the text that supposedly "taught a generation how to copulate."[75] In particular, consider how similar Van de Velde's description of normal marital "possession" is to Dworkin's:

> What both man and woman, driven by obscure primitive urges, wish to feel in the sexual act, is the essential force of *maleness*, which expresses itself in a sort of violent and absolute *possession* of the woman. And so both of them can and do exult in a certain degree of male aggression and dominance—whether actual or apparent—which proclaims this essential force.[76]

This book considers the possibility that women who have resisted the kind of "normality" described by Van de Velde—women who, in one way or another, have not measured up to the "possession" model of sexual intercourse—were often sent off to sex therapy for rehabilitation. There, they may have gone through various procedures, with different stages and instructions, different justifications and measures, all directed to the accomplishment of pleasure, autonomy, and marital harmony, but may have wound-up receiving something else. They may have come away with the understanding that it is their duty, as well as in their interests, to give their husband the kind of sexual experience he wants and expects. It is these possibilities that I will now attempt to bring into focus.

PART 1
SEX THERAPY PREHISTORY

1
Freud, Dora, and Compulsory Sexuality

> The fact is that whenever you are preoccupied with something, with some trouble or with some problem which is a big thing in your life—as sex is, for instance—then no matter what you start from, the association will lead finally and inevitably back to the same theme.
> —Ludwig Wittgenstein, "Conversations on Freud" (1966)

Freud never published a book or paper on vaginismus, he offered no hypotheses on how to treat patients experiencing sexual intercourse difficulties, and in fact showed little interest in the mechanics of copulation. He did, however, refocus the treatment of sexual disorders onto the patient's mind. As Foucault put it, "before Freud, one sought to localize sexuality as closely as possible: in sex, in its reproductive functions, in its immediate anatomical localizations; one fell back upon the biological minimum: organ, instinct, and finality."[1] After Freud, sex became linked to every imaginable social and psychological process: "It is no longer a question simply of saying what was done—the sexual act—and how it was done; but of reconstructing, in and around the act, the thoughts that recapitulated it, the obsessions that accompanied it, the images, desires, modulations, and quality of the pleasure that animated it."[2] Freud inspired psychoanalysts, psychiatrists, and Western culture in general to search out everything that had the faintest connection to sex. He did this by constituting sex as the secret, yet omnipresent, source of human motivation.[3] From a "shadow in a daydream," to the most fleeting feelings and behaviors, every human activity, for Freud, had a sexual dimension and therefore had to be exposed, studied, and understood in the most explicit terms.

As William Graham Cole described Freud's point of view, "everywhere he looked, he found libido, in all cultural achievement, in art, in friendship, in religion," and in everything his patients said.[4] At the same time, Freud trivialized and dismissed his patients' descriptions of nonsexual experience: Whether that patient was the "Wolf Man," the "Rat Man," or "Dora," he tried to convince them that at heart, whether they admitted it or not, they were driven by sexual desire. He compelled them to treat sexuality as their most powerful source of motivation.

In his papers on technique, Freud may have contended that a psychoanalyst should "turn his own unconscious like a receptive organ towards the transmitting unconscious of the patient. He must adjust himself to the patient as a telephone receiver is adjusted to the transmitting microphone,"[5] but in practice he was quite different. As a former patient of Freud's once remarked, "he would wait until he found an association which would fit into his scheme of interpretation and pick it up like a detective at a line-up who waits until he sees his man."[6] This is especially true with regard to Freud's management of Dora, which Steven Marcus described as positively demonic: "That *daimon* in whose service Freud knows no limits is the spirit of science, the truth, or 'reality'—it does not matter which. . . . Yet it must be emphasized the 'reality' Freud insists upon is very different from the 'reality' that Dora is claiming and clinging to."[7] Toril Moi also described Freud's management of Dora as fiercely one-sided, but for Moi, Freud's *daimon* is patriarchy: "Freud, for instance, systematically refuses to consider female sexuality as an active, independent drive. Again and again he exhorts Dora to accept herself as an object of Herr K."[8] For Jonathon Katz, Freud's *daimon* is heteronormativity, given his almost unwavering bias in favor of Dora's alleged sexual desire for her father and "Herr K.," in contrast to her alleged homoerotic feelings for "Frau K.," which Katz argued he denigrated as "a passing pubescent phase—a stage on the road to heterosexuality."[9] And for Claire Kahane, Freud's *daimon* is Freud himself, his own sexual desires, and his own need for acceptance and confirmation in the scientific community. Kahane argued that while Freud claimed he was focused on Dora's story, "what contemporary readings of Dora suggest is that, as brilliant as Freud was in constructing a narrative of Dora's desire, he essentially represented his own."[10] Whether Freud was indeed operating in the service of science, truth, reality, male privilege, heteronormativity, or his own needs—each of which, arguably, played a crucial role in his construction of Dora's story—my position here is that Freud was also operating as a *daimon* in the service of "compulsory sexuality," the idea that everyone harbors a profound and continuous need for sex.[11]

This chapter shows how Freud's "talking cure" not only replaced the surgeon's scalpel as the principal intermediary between a woman's body and medical standards of sexual normality, it shows how a therapist attempted to project his sexual interests onto a woman as a form of therapy. The chapter's overall goal is to construct a sort of conceptual model for examining how sex therapy may have harmed women in their capacity as knowers.[12] In the name of treating Dora's psychological symptoms, Freud bombarded her with sexual interpretations—confronting her, pursuing her, laying traps—all for the sake of drawing out admissions that reflected and supported his own erotic preoccupations.[13] Freud imposed his sexual story onto Dora, while simultaneously excluding, negating, and nullifying Dora's own thoughts, feelings, and experiential reality. And perhaps most important for the future of sex therapy, the chapter shows how Freud continuously rejected Dora's denial of sexual motivation.

Dora's Story—An Overview

The two main characters in Dora's story, apart from Dora and Freud, are her father, a wealthy industrialist who originally took her to Freud to consult about her persistent cough and hoarseness, and Herr K., a family friend who, on at least two occasions, tried to seduce Dora. Herr K.'s first sexual advance on Dora occurred when she was thirteen, at Herr K.'s office. There, he suddenly took her in his arms and kissed her on the lips. About two years later, Herr K. made another unwelcome sexual advance, at which time she slapped his face and hurried away.

Dora's treatment lasted only eleven weeks, from October through December, 1900.[14] At the conclusion of their penultimate session, after Freud had expressed satisfaction in the way he had interpreted her dreams, she "replied in a deprecatory tone: 'Why, has anything so very remarkable come out?'"[15] Then, at the beginning of the next session, she told him she was there for the last time.[16] Apparently fed up with his rude insinuations and aggressive manner, she had made up her mind "to put up with" the therapy only until the end of the year. In a postscript, Freud blamed the abrupt ending of Dora's treatment on himself, for failing to recognize that she had transferred her highly conflicted love for Herr K. onto her therapist.

Freud's Sexual Fixations

When Freud asked Dora about her relationship with Herr K., she told him that his initial seduction attempts had filled her with disgust, but Freud thought otherwise: "This was surely just the situation to call up a distinct feeling of sexual excitement in a girl of fourteen [thirteen][17] who had never before been approached."[18] Freud interpreted Dora's disgust as confirmation that she had actually been excited by Herr K. Such an interpretation—when Dora's outright denial of sexual feeling is treated as confirmatory evidence—raises the question of whether Freud was prepared to accept anything Dora said that contradicted his own sexual preoccupations. Was there any way she could disconfirm his sexual imputations and projections? Apparently not, because when Freud asked Dora if she recalled feeling Herr K.'s erection pressing against her leg during this encounter, and she responded in the negative, he insisted she must have, whether she knew it or not: "The perception was revolting to her; it was dismissed from her memory, repressed, and replaced by the innocent sensation of pressure upon her thorax, which in turn derived an excessive intensity from its repressed source."[19] The absence of Dora's confirmation not only had no discernible effect on Freud's conviction that Herr K. had an erection and that Dora had felt it press against her, Freud went so far as to claim, without one iota of evidence, that Dora became so sexually aroused by Herr K.'s erection, she experienced "an analogous change in the corresponding female organ, the clitoris."[20]

Freud believed that Dora had been profoundly attracted to Herr K., even though when he "informed her of this conclusion she did not assent to it."[21] Her lack of assent was simply dismissed. A few sentences later, Freud claimed a small victory when Dora's overt denial appeared to shift into something more equivocal. According to Freud, "when the quantity of material that had come up had made it difficult for her to persist in her denial," Dora admitted that at one point she "might" have been attracted Herr K.[22] Freud did not explain why he chose the conditional modal, "might," to convey Dora's assent, suggesting her uncertainty. But no matter: for Freud, the slightest, most ambiguous sign of Dora's acceptance of his sexual hypotheses was always treated as directly confirming, while any uncertainty about them was dismissed: "If a patient exhibits doubts in the course of his narrative, an empirical rule teaches us to disregard such expressions of his judgment entirely."[23]

At no point during Dora's treatment did she introduce the topic of her sexual feelings or interests, at no point did Freud take her denials of sexual feelings or interests seriously, and at no point did he suggest the feasibility of alternative, nonsexual explanations for her symptoms or behavior, even though such alternative explanations were always possible. It should not have been very difficult, for example, for Freud, or anyone else, to come up with a nonsexual explanation for an adolescent girl's intense interest in the small children she cares for. But for Freud, Dora's motive for babysitting Herr K.'s children had to have had an underlying sexual dimension: Dora's "preoccupation with his children was evidently a cloak for something else that Dora was anxious to hide from herself and from other people."[24] Similarly, it should not have been very difficult for Freud, or anyone else, to entertain the possibility that Dora had reacted to Herr K.'s advances with disgust, as well as a host of other negative feelings, such as shock, revulsion, and panic, seeing as she was, after all, only thirteen, and Herr K. was her father's age, the parent of two young children, and the husband of a close friend of hers. But Freud did not consider those possibilities. For him, no nonsexual reaction or motivation, however plausible or ordinary, can be compatible with "deep" interpersonal psychology.

A bit later in the text, Freud claimed that Dora "tacitly accepted" his explanation that her cough and the throat tickle that preceded it were caused by her unconscious wish to suck her father's penis. This, of course, raises the question of how Dora could "tacitly accept" Freud's interpretation of a wish he attributed to her unconscious. Nonetheless, he soldiered on, providing several reasons why he believed his interpretation of her sexual motivation was correct: The first is that, according to Freud, she was already quite aware that lovers sometimes engage in oral sex: "She knew very well, she said, that there was more than one way of obtaining sexual gratification,"[25] as if knowledge of a sex act supports the notion that one would fantasize such an act. The second is Freud's "rule" that a symptom represents a sexual fantasy. Thus, for Freud, "the conclusion was inevitable that with her spasmodic cough ... she pictured to herself a scene of [oral] sexual gratification,"[26] a conclusion, in other words, derived from an untested a priori rule and not from observations of Dora. The third is that Dora had a long history of oral sexual fixation: "She remembered very well that in her childhood she had been a 'suck-a-thumbs,'"[27] which raises the question, by what evidence did Freud classify Dora's infantile thumb-sucking as a precursor to adult genital behavior? What was the basis for this assertion other than his obsessive need to see evidence of sexual desire everywhere?[28] The fourth is that Dora complained again and again about her father's affair with Frau K., Herr K.'s wife. "I can think of nothing else," she had told Freud.[29] While children often respond badly to the discovery of a parent's extramarital affair for any number of reasons having nothing to do with sexuality (e.g., the parent's implied dishonesty, betrayal, immorality, etc.), Freud believed that Dora's repeated complaint about her father's affair could only indicate one thing: her wish to have sex with him. Freud's explanation reveals that for Freud the challenge was not to learn about Dora's experience but rather to retell her story in a way that emphasized (and affirmed) the narrative coherence of his own sexual fixations, in this case, his belief in children's sexual attraction to their parents:

> I have learnt to look upon unconscious love relations like this (which may be recognized by their abnormal consequences)—between a father and a daughter, or between a mother and a son—as a revival of germs of feeling in infancy. I have shown at length elsewhere at what an early age sexual attraction makes itself felt between parents and children, and I have explained that the myth of Oedipus is probably to be regarded as a poetical rendering of what is typical in these relations. Distinct traces are probably to be found in most people of an early partiality of this kind—on the part of the daughter for the father, or on the part of a son for the mother.[30]

When Freud shared his conclusion with Dora that she was "completely in love" with her father, he wrote, "She of course gave me her usual reply: 'I don't remember that,'" a denial Freud immediately dismissed based on Dora, soon after, telling him the story of a seven-year-old girl who hated her mother, wished her dead, and wanted to marry her father.[31] From these comments Freud drew the inference that his sexual hypothesis about Dora was correct. His reason: "I am in the habit of regarding associations such as this, which bring forward something that agrees with the content of an assertion of mine, as a confirmation from the unconscious of what I have said."[32] Freud's very next sentence is telling: "No other kind of 'Yes' can be extracted from the unconscious; there is no such thing at all as an unconscious 'No.'"[33] It is telling because it makes the denial of sexual motivation impossible. For even if a patient were to explicitly and forcefully reject such motivation, Freud could still say that on an unconscious level a "no" equals a "yes." Thus, in 1923, in a note added to his original study of Dora, Freud asserted:

> There is another very remarkable and entirely trustworthy form of confirmation from the unconscious, which I had not recognized at the time this was written: namely, an exclamation on the part of the patient of "I didn't think that," or "I didn't think of that." This can be translated point-blank into: "Yes, I was unconscious of that."[34]

When Freud told Dora that she felt "obliged to summon up her infantile affection for her father and exaggerate it, in order to protect herself against the feelings of love [for Herr K.] which were constantly pressing forward into consciousness," Dora's response was "a most emphatic negative."[35] Again, this did not discourage Freud in the least for the reason that

> The "No" uttered by a patient after a repressed thought has been presented to his conscious perception for the first time does no more than register the existence of a repression and its severity; it acts, as it were, as a gauge of the repression's strength. If this "No," instead of being regarded as an expression of an impartial judgment (of which, indeed, the patient is incapable), is ignored, and if work is continued, the first evidence soon begins to appear that in such case "No" signifies the desired "Yes."[36]

What this means, for Freud, is that the more strongly Dora, or any other patient, insists that an experience has nothing to do with sexual desire, the more obvious it becomes that it does.

Dora's Dreams

The only parts of Dora's case study where Freud quotes her at length are the dream interpretation sections. What is most important to notice there is that in each of the two dreams Dora shared with Freud, her words, if taken at face value, provide no hint of sexual feelings. They are entirely nonsexual. Yet by the time Freud finished interpreting them, they had become saturated with sexuality. Consider, for example, how she described her first dream:

> A house was on fire. My father was standing beside my bed and woke me up. I dressed myself quickly. Mother wanted to stop and save her jewel-case; but father said: "I refuse to let myself and my two children be burnt for the sake of your jewel-case." We hurried downstairs, and as soon as I was outside I woke up.[37]

Freud transformed this apparently nonsexual dream into one entirely focused on Dora's sexual wishes. To begin, he asked Dora where and when she had the dream, to which she answered that she had it at the place where Herr K. had attempted to seduce her and that it occurred after the seduction attempt. Freud found this illuminating and told Dora: "Now I am certain that the dream was an immediate effect of your experience with Herr K."[38] Freud did not ask Dora if his observation was correct; he simply asserted that it was, a pattern that prevailed throughout the interpretation of both of Dora's dreams.

After she informed him that Herr K. had once given her a jewel case as a gift, he jumped to the conclusion that the jewel case in Dora's dream represented a clear and utterly embarrassing sexual connection to Herr K.: "Perhaps you do not know that 'jewel-case' [Schmuckkastchen] is a favourite expression for the same thing that you alluded to not long ago by means of the reticule you were wearing—for the female genitals, I mean."[39] Dora's reaction: "I knew you would say that," suggests her frustration over Freud's one-track mind, her perception that no matter what she brought up, whether a dream or some problem in her life, his interpretations would lead finally and inevitably back to the same theme—sex. However, in keeping with Freud's belief that a patient's "no" can only mean an unconscious "yes," he treated her comment, "I knew you would say that," as totally confirmatory. Freud's response to Dora not only illustrates how, for Freud, Dora's voice in the assignment of her motivations had been rendered mute, but also how Freud constructed Dora's wish to copulate with Herr K. solely from his own imagination, for his own purposes, without showing any concern for how his construction appealed to her:

> The meaning of the dream is now becoming even clearer. . . . Now bring your mind back to the jewel-case which Herr K. gave you. You have there the starting point for a parallel line of thoughts, in which Herr K. is to be put in the place of your father just as he was in the matter of standing beside your bed. He gave you a jewel-case; so you are to give him your jewel-case. That was why I spoke just now of a "return-present." . . . So you are ready to give Herr K. what his wife

withholds from him. That is the thought which has had to be repressed with so much energy, and which has made it necessary for every one of its elements to be turned into its opposite. The dream confirms once more what I had already told you before you dreamed it—that you are summoning up your old love for your father in order to protect yourself against your love for Herr K. But what do all these efforts show? Not only that you are afraid of Herr K., but that you are still more afraid of yourself, and of the temptation you feel to yield to him. In short, these efforts prove once more how deeply you loved him."[40]

Freud did not quote Dora's reaction to this interpretation, but he did comment, dismissively, that "naturally Dora would not follow me in this part of the interpretation."[41] Perhaps if Freud had said to Dora, "It is an interesting coincidence that Herr K. gave you a jewel case as a gift and that you dreamed of a jewel case at the very site you met with him," she might have followed him. But Freud went much farther. He said that the jewel case in her dream represents her genitals and reveals that Dora was ready to reward Herr K. with a "return-present"— sexual intercourse—proving "once more how deeply" she loved him. Here, as in all of Freud's other explanations of Dora's sexual motivations, there is not a single example of Dora's straightforward agreement. Nor is there any direct evidence that Dora was attracted to Herr K. Why then did Freud insist that she was? The simplest answer is that he was not interested in her agreement. He only wanted to tell her story to his own satisfaction, in a manner that conformed to his own sexual biases and preoccupations.

A Masturbation Interrogation

At one point during Freud's interpretation of Dora's "house-on-fire" dream, when he was trying to understand why her father had been unhappy that her brother's room had no separate entrance, Dora said, "Something might happen in the night so that it might be necessary to leave the room."[42] This made Freud think of children's bed-wetting, an association that prompted him to try what he called "a little experiment." As part of his scheme to make Dora confess that she used to wet her bed as a child, he asked her to look around his office to see if she noticed anything special about a table on which he had placed a match stand. She did not notice it. Then he pointed it out to her and asked if she had any idea why parents warn their children to never play with matches. "On account of the risk of fire," Dora answered. "Not on that account," said Freud, correcting her. "They are warned not to 'play with fire,' and a particular belief is associated with the warning." Dora still did not know what he was getting at. "Very well, then," Freud finally told her. "The fear is that if they do they will wet the bed. The antithesis of 'water' and 'fire' must be the bottom of this. Perhaps it is believed that they will dream of fire and then try and put it out with water."[43] This, in connection with Dora's recollection of her father waking her up in her dream to save her from the fire, prompted Freud to tell Dora that she had been "addicted to bed-wetting up to a later age than is usual with children."[44] Dora hesitated at first, but then said that she did recall wetting her bed "for some time" and that "it must have been serious because I remember now that the doctor was called in."[45] For Freud, this admission confirmed that she had been a masturbator. He was sure based on his prior understanding that Dora's father had been suffering from syphilis, coupled with Dora sharing her belief that "she too was suffering from a venereal disease." When Dora said "that she was afflicted with catarrh (leucorrhoea)," any doubts Freud had about Dora's masturbatory history disappeared.[46] Why would catarrh (vaginal discharge) indicate masturbation? Freud's incredibly vague explanation was that "all the other causes which were commonly assigned to that complaint were put in the background by masturbation."[47] After Freud put the pieces of this edifice together, he told Dora that "she was now on the way to finding an answer to her own question of why it was precisely *she* had fallen ill—by confessing that she had masturbated, probably in childhood."[48]

Not surprisingly, Dora refused to go along. She flatly denied his accusation. But at this point, it had become clear that it didn't make any difference whether Dora "confessed" or not. The greater issue was that Freud was unwilling and unable to hear her, and, as we will see in the next chapter, an entire generation of women would soon be receiving the same kind of discursive reception as part of their sex therapy. Thus, Freud remained convinced that Dora had been a masturbator, despite her denials, and proceeded to add additional pieces of evidence aimed at "tearing" this admission from her, an effort he began a few days after she confessed to bed-wetting as a child.

That is when he noticed that she wore at her waist a small reticule: "As she lay on the sofa and talked, she kept playing with it—opening it, putting a finger into it, shutting it again."[49] Then, after silently watching her touch her reticule for a few moments, he opened up, accusing her of symbolically masturbating in his office. For Janet Malcolm, in this moment, it was as if Freud had said to Dora, "Aha! I know about you. I know your dirty little secrets.... Look at what you're doing now as you lie there playing with your reticule—opening it, putting a finger into it, shutting it again!"[50] Freud did not include Dora's immediate response to this accusation, although one can imagine she was shocked and mortified. The only comment he attributed to her was, "Why should I not wear a reticule like this, as it is now the fashion to do?"[51] Characteristically, Dora's unwillingness to go along with Freud's interpretation had no effect on him. He remained certain he had hit a bullseye and thus went on to write that "Dora's reticule, which came apart at the top in the usual way, was nothing but a representation of the genitals, and her playing with it, her opening it and putting her finger in it, was an entirely unembarrassed yet unmistakable pantomimic announcement of what she would like to do with them—namely, to masturbate."[52]

Freud added one more piece of evidence to use against Dora. On the day that she brought her "house-on-fire" dream to him, as he entered his consultation room, he noticed that she hurriedly concealed a letter she had been reading. When he asked her whom the letter was from, she at first refused to say. Soon after, she told him it was from her grandmother and had nothing to do with her treatment. This gave Freud the idea that "Dora only wanted to play 'secrets' with me, and to hint that she was on the point of allowing her secret to be torn from her by the physician."[53] The secret, of course, was that she had been a masturbator, a conclusion he defended in the language of a prosecutor making a summation to the jury:

> The reproaches against her father for having made her ill, together with the self-reproach underlying them, the leucorrhoea, the playing with the reticule, the bed-wetting after her sixth year, the secret she would not allow the physicians to *tear from her—the circumstantial evidence of her having masturbated in childhood seems to me complete and without a flaw.*[54]

Carl Jung long ago noted that Freud was obsessed with sexuality. Whenever Freud spoke on the topic, his "tone would become urgent, almost anxious ... a strange deeply moved expression came over his face"[55] Jung could not explain Freud's strange attitude, except to say that "there was no mistaking the fact that Freud was emotionally involved with his sexual theory to an extraordinary degree."[56]

What makes Freud's sexual preoccupation culturally significant is that it was not seen as his peculiarity, or at least not only as his peculiarity. Rather, it was widely perceived by scholars, physicians, and literati as a transformative discovery, revolutionary and freeing, comparable to the achievements of Copernicus, Darwin, and Einstein. Before Freud, sexuality had been perceived as an optional, low-level topic of conversation, but after, it came to be viewed as necessary—the very foundation of life. As Alfred Kazin put it, "until Freud, novelists and dramatists had never dared to think that science would back up their belief that personal passion is a stronger force in people's lives than socially accepted morality. Thanks to Freud, these insights now form a widely shared body of knowledge."[57] More recently, Peter Tatchell summed up Freud's influence as "an emancipatory understanding of sexual desire"; by bringing "this vast range of sexual expression to public attention and scientific understanding, and asserting its often commonplace occurrence, Freud struck a major blow against the denials and strictures of puritan morality."[58]

The problem, of course, is that, oftentimes, denials of sexual experience and sexual motivation have nothing to do with puritan morality or psychological repression. Many are completely truthful. As we have learned in recent years from the emerging discourses on asexuality, numerous people do not experience sexual desire.[59] Numerous others experience sexual desire at times, but only selectively and mildly, and many feel more motivated by nonsexual types of feeling such as friendship.[60] Indeed, if we assume that human sexual variation is continuous and diverse and not merely bimodal—not merely sexual or nonsexual—then we can begin to appreciate how many people have been and can be misrepresented by the Freudian compulsion to read sex into all human activity.[61]

What is most troubling here, and what makes Freud's "Dora" most significant for the development of the sex therapy profession, is that in treating Dora's accounts of nonsexual experience as false and meaningless, as so much cover for her "true" sexual feelings, Freud not only subjected Dora to his own vision of sexuality, he not only replaced her narrative with his, but he also showed an entire generation of physicians, psychologists, and other types of therapists how to do the same with their patients. Thanks to Freud and his management of Dora, the next generation of therapists had a conceptual framework for informing their patients that what they want and need on an unconscious level, despite their protests to the contrary and despite all objective evidence, is sex—masculine sex.

2
The Frigidity Epidemic

> Whenever a woman is incapable of achieving orgasm via coitus, provided the husband is an adequate partner, and prefers clitoral stimulation to any other form of sexual activity, she can be regarded as suffering from frigidity and requires psychiatric assistance.
> —Frank S. Caprio, *The Sexually Adequate Female* (1953)

Freud's belief that people have an omnipresent and innate need for sex, as demonstrated by the Dora study, led to one of sex therapy's organizing metaphors—the metaphor of the continuously flowing stream of sexual energy—the idea that psychological problems occur when an individual's sexual energy or libido behaves like "a stream whose main bed has been blocked."[1] According to Freud, the blocked stream "proceeds to fill up collateral channels which may hitherto have been empty," producing neuroses, inhibitions, and/or perversions.[2]

Widespread acceptance of this idea suggests why, during the second third of the twentieth century, psychoanalytically trained physicians focused so much attention on women's sexual reticence or "frigidity." For them, a woman with a blockage in her stream of sexual energy may appear uninterested in having sex (with her husband), but that is only the surface manifestation of the problem. As Vienna-trained psychiatrist Edmund Bergler explained to one of his patients, "Personality and symptoms are interconnected. Every time we talk about your wish to be rejected, refused, disappointed, we are talking about your frigidity."[3] Thus, in 1954, Bergler and a colleague Eduard Hitschmann claimed that the sexual frigidity problem is so widespread that it amounted to an "emotional plague."[4] In the words of psychiatrist Marie N. Robinson, whose book on women's sexual frigidity, *The Power of Sexual Surrender* (1959), sold over a million copies, "no other public health problem of our time even approaches this magnitude,"[5] a rather curious assessment since only a few decades earlier, coolness and reticence had been regarded as natural in women.[6] It is also curious since no comparable claim was being made with regard to men's sexual reticence, as if gynecologists and psychiatrists had never heard women complain that their husbands lacked sexual interest.[7] Indeed, concern over women's sexual frigidity so penetrated mainstream medicine during the 1940s and 1950s, that in 1950, the *Journal of the American Medical Association* published an article that began with the claim that "frigidity is one of the most common problems in gynecology. Gynecologists and psychiatrists, especially, are aware that perhaps 75 percent of all women derive little or no pleasure from the sexual act."[8]

To be sure, not all physicians at this time were thinking the same way about frigidity. For example, in 1950, physician Mary Mann Gillett, in her article, "Normal Frigidity in Women: A Plea to the Family Physician," argued that women were often disinclined to have sex with their husbands, not because of their deep psychological problems, but because of their husband's rude, thoughtless behavior. Gillett wrote that "no scientific person" could claim that 75% of all Americans are frigid, as the authors of the JAMA article did.[9] And five years later, an anonymous JAMA reviewer for John F. Oliven's *Sexual Hygiene and Pathology*, echoed Gillett's stance, saying, "It is absurd to call the most passionate women frigid simply because they cannot achieve orgasm in normal intercourse."[10]

To situate Freud in this discourse, he may have been the "father of the vaginal orgasm,"[11] as Ann Koedt called him, and he may have been the architect of the theoretical structures underlying the new conceptualization of frigidity—namely, that everyone has an inborn well-spring of sexual energy and that women's sexual development is far more complicated and precarious than men's, since only women must exchange sexual zones (from clitoris to vagina) and primary love objects (from mother to father). But Freud was not very interested in sexual frigidity, per se. He wrote very little on the topic, and when he did, it was with pronounced hesitation, as in this excerpt from his *Introductory Lecture* on femininity:

> The sexual frigidity of women ... is a phenomenon that is still insufficiently understood. Sometimes it is psychogenic and in that case accessible to influence; but in other cases it suggests the hypothesis of its being constitutionally determined and even of there being a contributory anatomical factor.[12]

By contrast, Edmund Bergler, and a host of other psychoanalytically trained physicians, showed no hesitation. Unlike Freud, they were not speculating on the possibility of women's frigidity; they were not attempting to refine their understanding. Rather, they were spreading the doctrine that women's neuroses in their many and complex manifestations can be reduced to a single measurable disease process—frigidity:

> The consequences of frigidity are tragic for the woman. They lead from dissatisfaction, depression, hysterical symptoms, to the typical defense mechanism—denial by the woman that she is ill and constant changing of husbands and male friends.[13]

This chapter examines how physicians and other sex therapists documented such claims. Reading medical texts as accounts, I focus on how mid-twentieth century Freudians saw, described, and explained frigidity in their case studies and in writings for the general public in sex guides, marriage manuals, and advice columns. As Freudian therapists persuaded themselves and others that sexual frigidity represents a public health threat of the first magnitude, they represented men and their sexuality as the norm, and women and their sexuality as suspect, in need of the most rigorous surveillance and control.

The New Definition

Before the middle portion of the twentieth century, frigidity had always been understood as a semantically fluid concept variously referring to a deficiency in a woman's sexual desire or a deficiency in her capacity for sexual arousal and/or orgasm, or some combination thereof.[14] However, in their landmark text, *Frigidity in Women*, Eduard Hitschmann and Edmund Bergler (1936) defined frigidity in substantially more rigid, inflexible terms:

> It is no matter whether the woman is aroused during coitus or remains cold, whether the excitement is weak or strong, whether it breaks off at the beginning or the end, slowly or suddenly, whether it is dissipated in preliminary acts, or has been lacking from the beginning. The sole criterion of frigidity is the absence of the *vaginal* orgasm.[15]

The first effect of this definitional shift was to enlarge the reach of sex therapy. Under the new definition, frigidity no longer meant simply disinterest in sex. As Bergler explained, no longer did the definition extend only to the woman whose sexual attitude is entirely negative, who "constantly reiterates that the procedure is dirty and disgusting, and feels disgust if 'subjected' to 'that ordeal.'"[16] Now it included the woman who feels sexually responsive, who enjoys "preliminary acts" and phases of coitus, "even reaching clitoridean orgasm during these manipulations."[17] Under the new definition, a state of semi-arousal did not constitute a woman as semi-responsive or semi-normal. It constituted her as frigid and neurotic.

What's more, diagnostic confirmation did not have to wait till all the information was in. All a physician needed was a hunch. He could make the frigidity diagnosis without even hearing a woman's side of the story. Consider, for example, how Bergler managed to label a patient's wife as frigid, sight unseen. The husband, whom Bergler called a "big businessman," had been married twenty-three years, and sought Bergler's help for his "premature ejaculation" problem.

When Bergler asked him how long intercourse usually lasted, the businessman answered, "approximately 30 to 40 minutes."[18] Bergler responded by congratulating the man on his potency and then acquainted him with the "empirical fact" that typical intercourse lasts only two to three minutes. Bergler went on to say that this "patient had understood as premature ejaculation his inability to protract intercourse until his wife's orgasm came. Since she reached one, seldom enough, only after an hour, she accused him of having premature ejaculation."[19] When Bergler assured his patient that he did not suffer from premature ejaculation, the businessman jumped to his feet in triumph. Berger asked him to return to his seat to inform him that he suffered from "something worse." This "worse" diagnosis, Bergler explained, was his "pathologic masochistic attachment to his frigid wife, who made him swallow all this nonsense for a quarter of a century, exploited him financially on a grand scale and induced in him a strong feeling of guilt because of his alleged sexual inadequacy."[20]

According to Hitschmann's and Bergler's new definition of frigidity, "every woman is frigid if she is incapable of reaching vaginal orgasm during the sex act quite independently of whether she is aroused during the act,"[21] meaning that even women who appear to take pleasure in intercourse could be swept into the frigidity net. Thus, Bergler asked readers to "imagine a beautiful, coquettish woman, with a great deal of natural, and still more artificial, charm. At first glance, she impresses one as being thoroughly womanly, the personification of 'sex appeal.' Everything about her revolves around sexuality; every word and every glance seem to be sexual challenges to men."[22] However, she is not the person she appears to be. When the physician peers behind her erotic façade, he discovers "that she is full of unconscious hatred of the man, whom she cannot forgive for the very fact of being a man," which, as far as Hitschmann and Bergler were concerned, settled the question of her frigidity.[23] Much as Freud defined thirteen-year-old Dora as hysterical for registering disgust when Herr K., a married man more than twice her age, tried to kiss her, Hitschmann and Bergler believed that any woman who refused her husband's sexual advances had to be both hysterical and frigid, since, in their eyes, "hysterical women are without exception frigid."[24]

While Hitschmann, Bergler, and other physicians who advanced the new frigidity narrative never stated that all women are frigid, they found hints and premonitions of this disease in virtually all their women patients. Because they defined frigidity in negative terms—as the absence of vaginal orgasm—they required little for proof, and almost anything could arouse suspicion. For instance, in 1969, a woman wrote to psychiatrist-psychoanalyst Renatus Hartogs, advice columnist for *Cosmopolitan*, with a seemingly innocuous concern: She did not feel "overpowering desire" for her boyfriend, she could not match his level of sexual interest, and when he tried to make love to her, she sometimes needed some kind of stimulation "to be made excited."[25] She concluded her letter with the question, "Is something the matter with me?" Hartogs's answer was an unequivocal *yes*. She had to be frigid. As far as Hartogs was concerned, it was obvious that she had difficulty relinquishing "inner controls" and needed to consider the possibility that she was using "sex as a weapon to dominate or disappoint the male." Despite the fact that the letter-writer never mentioned her childhood or parental relationships, Hartogs[26] suggested that the explanation for her lack of sexual interest was her "unhappy and disturbing childhood experiences and an unfavorable parent-child relationship," which, he concluded, had the unfortunate effect of making her "suspicious of the male . . . of his urges and intentions."[27]

A Master Lens

Among the many case studies illustrating psychoanalytic approaches to frigidity at mid-twentieth century, I found none in which the patient first complained of frigidity, but after her history had been scrutinized, the problem turned out to be something else. This is partly because psychoanalysis, as a treatment method, is not usually focused on a specific symptom. Ideally, people go into analysis to explore their whole personality. It should not be surprising, then, that in most of the psychoanalytic case studies dating from this period, patients began treatment with multiple presenting complaints other than frigidity. What did surprise me is that as treatment progressed, frigidity emerged as the central concern. For instance, Hitschmann and Bergler described a woman who came to treatment for help with depression and "a serious work inhibition." She was not seeking to increase her sexual desire for her husband. In fact, she was looking for ways to detach herself from him: she wanted to improve her chances of holding onto her job, which she hoped would give her "pecuniary independence and therefore the means to leave." Hitschmann and Bergler, however, traced her wish to end her marriage to her own sexual psychopathology: "The analysis showed that the patient confirmed and enjoyed masochistically the sadism of her husband who had built up an altogether subtle system of moral torment. Significantly, the patient was entirely frigid with her husband; her satisfaction lay in the enjoyment of anxiety pleasure, beside which there was also a strong need for punishment."[28]

Other patients described by Hitschmann and Bergler came for help with a wide variety of problems—animal phobias, neurotic forebodings, promiscuity, infidelity, homosexual wishes, agoraphobia, obsessive fears—but for each, in time, the analysis revealed the underlying dynamic as frigidity. Much as Heraclitus constituted fire as the material foundation for all things, Hitschmann and Bergler turned frigidity into a simple, yet primitive explanation for women's every neurotic complaint: Was the patient frustrated in her efforts to escape her husband, or was she frustrated in her efforts to get closer to him? Was she a nymphomaniac? Sexually overactive or sexually underactive? Nervous? Phobic? Depressed? Listless? An alcoholic? A man hater? A compulsive personality or a multiple personality? In each instance, Hitschmann and Bergler traced these problems to a single source—frigidity.[29]

Consider how Marie N. Robinson, a psychiatrist who specialized in the treatment of sexual frigidity, performed such a distillation on Molly, a patient who entered treatment after she had aborted two unwanted pregnancies, the second resulting in a urinary infection that required hospitalization. While Molly did not identify herself as frigid and was not seeking help with problems of sexual arousal or desire, Robinson was impressed by the fact that her new patient had recently begun an affair with an impoverished art student who, she surmised, "obviously had no real feeling for Molly and . . . no real ability to care for any other person." Robinson was also impressed by the fact that Molly's orgasmic history seemed limited to forbidden and guilty acts "with a person who was, in her mind, anathema to her parents. . . . For if a man was respectable, 'meant well by her,' loved her, in her unconscious life she would immediately associate him with her parents and their approval, and this would kill all sexual feeling in her. She would be frigid with him."[30]

This, then, is how Freudian psychiatrists turned frigidity into an epidemic: not only by seeing signs of the disease where their patients did not, but also by portraying sexual health in impossibly stringent and contradictory terms. To become sexually liberated in the Freudian narrative, Molly had to curb and focus her sexuality. To overcome one "pathological inhibition," she had to embrace a whole set of new inhibitions, including rejection of sex with socially inappropriate partners. Orgasms outside marriage, whether vaginal or clitoral, indicated frigidity.[31] She also had to abandon her clitoris, defined by Freudians as a tiny—and painfully inadequate—version of the male phallus. This "rudimentary" organ, according to psychoanalyst Marie Bonaparte, is "never destined to achieve, even in its owner's imagination, the degree of activity to which the penis can lay claim, for in this respect the male organ is far better endowed by nature."[32] A woman who enjoys sensation in her clitoris, who regards her clitoris the way men regard their penis—a "clitoridal woman"—was seen as butch, masculine, and destined to be dissatisfied. As Lundberg and Farnham explained in *Modern Woman; the Lost Sex* (1947), "the woman's unconscious wish to herself possess the organ upon which she must depend militates greatly against her ability to accept its vast power to satisfy her when proffered to her in love."[33] Such women, according to Dr. Maurice Chideckel in *Female Sex Perversion* (1935), "talk and act like men, become more masculine than feminine, and are therefore frigid. They have no desire for copulation, never think of it; and when they do have physical union enjoy no sensation of pleasure. To them sexuality is superfluous."[34]

If it can be said that Freudian psychoanalysis traditionally interprets patients' stories as never finished—one life event or symbol interpreted through a second, a second through a third, a third through a fourth, and so on, each narrative coloring the next in an endless chain of signification—then it can be said that mid-twentieth century psychoanalysis reversed that interpretive scheme, as patients' stories came to a sudden stop as soon as any sign of frigidity emerged. Thus, everything became accessible, with nothing left to interpret or analyze, when another patient, Patricia, told Dr. Robinson, as reported in *The Power of Sexual Surrender*, that her husband's body appeared "skinny, white, and ugly, with an enormous penis. It was as if he were nothing but a big disgusting sex organ," so offensive that "she could feel no tenderness or warmth—she could not even simulate it."[35] Forget the possibility that the husband may have been "cruel, selfish, demanding, and insensitive to her needs," just as Patricia described him.[36] Forget the possibility that he may have been physically repulsive. The critical point is that through the frigidity lens, Patricia was repelled by her husband not because something about him called forth that response; she was repelled because of her pre-existing frigidity.

Women Are to Blame

Earlier discourses on frigidity would have reached very different conclusions about Molly and Patricia. For instance, Theodor Van de Velde (1926) interpreted sexual frigidity as innate in women and as relatively natural. In his words, "inadequate sensibility in coitus at the beginning of active sexual life must be accounted physiologically normal in women: they have to learn to feel voluptuous pleasure and actual orgasm."[37] Since a woman's passivity is "innate," and therefore normal, her sexual response, according to Marie Bonaparte (1935), "always depends . . . upon the potency of her partner and especially upon the time he allows for gratification, which is usually achieved more slowly than his own."[38] From Havelock Ellis's (1926) perspective, "the fact that a woman remains cool in the embrace of a man, or even in the embrace of several men successively, does not prove that she is not capable of strong sexual feeling; it only shows that these men were unable to awaken her sexual feeling."[39] As gynecologist Robert Latou Dickinson put it, "it takes two persons to make one frigid woman."[40]

Such assessments, however, carried little weight with mid-twentieth century Freudians. In fact, they were seen as dangerously misleading, first, because "by declaring vaginal frigidity 'normal,' the neurosis hiding behind this symptom is overlooked . . . preventing medical scrutiny and treatment."[41] Second, by stressing the man's failure to awaken his wife's sexual feeling as the explanation for her coolness, they seemed to confuse cause with effect. As Bergler put it, "the greatest Casanova is helpless against frigidity. It is not to be cured by tricks or by some special art of lovemaking."[42] Even when the man is impotent, he is not responsible for his wife's frigidity: "One must never forget that the coldness of the woman has an influence on the potency of the man. A sexually rejecting behavior on the part of the woman can call forth a psychic indifference toward her, even in a healthy man."[43]

Psychiatrist Frank Caprio (1953) wrote, "Few women realize that men are sexually sensitive. The penis may be merely an appendage of flesh but it has a 'soul' as it were. When insulted it behaves accordingly."[44] Caprio went on to explain how many frigid wives, through an inconsiderate word or action, force their husbands to go on "sexual strike."[45] To illustrate, he shared the story of a man who attended a party with his wife where an attractive young woman approached in a flirtatious fashion and sat on his lap. This so outraged his wife that she slapped him across the face in front of everyone. A few weeks later, after she apologized, the husband attempted to put the incident behind him, but when he tried to resume sexual relations with her, he discovered that he could not perform. Caprio had no doubt as to the cause of the trouble: the husband had been "psychically castrated by his wife." He wanted to have intercourse with her, he did his best, but finally, in desperation, divorced her "and married some other woman with whom he was sexually potent. His former wife never remarried and still regrets her costly mistake."[46]

Caprio's story has three morals. The first is that a woman is responsible should her husband leave her for another woman, the second is that a woman has the capacity to make otherwise healthy men impotent, and the third is that a woman has only herself to blame if she cannot function in a sexually healthy way. From Bergler's vantage point, "nothing is more laughable and, if you will, more tragic than a potent husband who believes he is responsible for his wife's frigidity."[47] This is because a man looks upon his wife's frigidity from a position of "absolutely stupid naivete," a position the wife herself sustains through an almost endless series of manipulations and lies. Proof of this can be found in the consultation room "where a woman who begins treatment for frigidity . . . begs the therapist not to mention her frigidity to her husband who believes that she is beginning a cure for "general nervousness." Proof can also be found in the bedroom where "a great number of frigid women pretend . . . to be satisfied, even after completely unsatisfactory intercourse."[48] They "maintain this illusion of enjoying sex vaginally by holding the thighs closely together . . . or they pretend to be highly excited, producing acrobatic movements."[49] Or, just as often, they blame their failure to become sexually aroused on their husband, as did one of Bergler's patients, Mrs. H., when she described her husband as a "block of ice," completely lacking in tenderness, unwilling to give her as much as a kiss or loving glance.[50] When Bergler met with Mr. H. to assess the merits of his patient's complaints, he found a man who "gave the impression of being under court-martial. He was tense, his features frozen."

> "What about your alleged lack of tenderness?" Bergler asked.
> "I hate the word," Mr. H. answered bitterly. "I get it as a reproach, served for breakfast and dinner—it's my good luck that I don't take lunch at home. My wife's first word after awakening, her last one before going to bed, has something to do with that damned tenderness. It drives me crazy."
> "Do you consider yourself a tender person?"
> "I don't know any more what the word means," he replied. "My wife uses it as a whip."[51]

What message does this dialogue convey? First, the woman is a shrew; the man, a sacrificial lamb. Pretending to be seeking tenderness, she nagged, demanded, and criticized, until she finally obtained what she unconsciously desired: a sexless marriage. Second, the woman cannot be trusted. She portrayed herself as her husband's victim without acknowledging her role in creating her bloodless, benumbed block of ice, a style of reportage Bergler found characteristic of frigid women, in general. According to him, women suffering from an inability to experience vaginal orgasm can be expected to employ the most artful alibis and excuses in shifting blame onto their spouse (e.g., "My husband has no respect for me as a lady. He asks me to use obscene words in bed."[52] "Normal sex has no attraction for my husband. He asks for all kinds of perversions, claiming I'm a neurotic fool for refusing." "My husband constantly reproaches me with frigidity. He just wants to be seduced and has no conception that civilized sex and 'jungle rape' are two different things." "My husband derives some vicarious pleasure from making all kinds of sexy allusions in the presence of our friends . . . as if I were the sexual property of his friends too."[53]). Yet, according to Bergler, it never occurs "to any of them to ask themselves why they chose their neurotic husband in the first place, or how they accounted for their own frigidity."[54] As psychiatrist Marie Robinson summed up, "the chief characteristic of women with this type of problem is evasiveness."[55] Women suffering from frigidity cannot be trusted to tell their story; their physicians and husbands have to tell their story for them, a phenomenon Miranda Fricker called "hermeneutical inequality"—when "the subject is rendered unable to make communicatively intelligible something which it is particularly in his or her interests to be able to render intelligible."[56]

For physicians, the diagnostic problem posed by frigid women's presumed lack of trustworthiness is easy enough to understand. If frigid women cannot be taken at their word, if they cannot be trusted to give an honest straightforward account of their sexual arousal, their frigidity has to be assigned on the basis of some other, more reliable source. For this reason, mid-twentieth century

Freudians proposed the manual examination of women's vaginal canal during their alleged orgasm.

As Hitschmann and Bergler insisted, "the only objective sign of frigidity is absence of *involuntary* muscular contraction in the pelvic region during female orgasm."[57] To test this hypothesis, gynecologist William S. Kroger performed an experiment on a prostitute, Miss G. C., who claimed she could deceive her clients into believing she was having a vaginal orgasm by voluntarily contracting her pelvic and perineal muscles. Kroger inserted a Kegel perinometer into her vagina and, after she was asked to simulate orgasm, found that she was indeed able to move the needle up thirty to forty points at will. However, when Kroger inserted his fingers into the depths of her vagina, and again asked her to simulate orgasm, he found "she had no ability to contract the deeper vaginal muscles."[58] While this appeared to confirm the Hitschmann–Bergler hypothesis, it opened another, related question: If measuring the contractions of the deeper vaginal muscles during coitus with one's fingers constitutes the final test of frigidity, then how are physicians to make these observations? How can they gain access to an area so private, at a moment so personal?

The answer turned out to be simple, almost obvious. Bergler and Kroger argued that access could be facilitated through the cooperation of the patient's husband: "These contractions are felt in the part of the penis deepest in the vagina; hence vaginal orgasm can readily be ascertained by the male during the sex act provided he is aware of this fact."[59] This led physicians to recommend that in cases where the frigidity diagnosis is in doubt, the doctor should "make inquiries of the husband as to the wife's response. He may help the husband to understand his wife's predicament by pointing out that in only one thing is the wife completely helpless, and that is in controlling the involuntary contractions of the pelvic and perineal muscles which occur at the end of coitus."[60]

What did physicians gain by enlisting the husband's cooperation in this way? They gained direct access to women's unfiltered sexual responses, which means that physicians and husbands could together define women, supervise them, and neutralize any impulse to deceive. As Bergler put it, "a man can be deceived by a clever woman in many things—in love, sensitivity, sexual interest, pleasure in intercourse. In only one thing is she helpless—the production of involuntary contractions."[61]

Measuring Frigidity

Once a woman had been identified as lacking involuntary contractions of the deeper vaginal muscles, the next step was to locate her frigidity on a scale, the highest grade being "total frigidity with vaginal anesthesia" where "the woman is wholly without sexual interest during intercourse."[62] One grade lower, "total frigidity with vaginal hypesthesia," describes the woman who has "slight excitement at the beginning of coitus" and "very slight sensitivity of the clitoris." Hitschmann and Bergler referred to the next grade as "relative frigidity with vaginal hypesthesis" characterized by "slight excitement throughout the act," which was followed by a fourth grade, "relative frigidity with vaginal sensitivity," consisting of "rising excitement" but with no orgasm. In a fifth grade, "clitoric orgasm with vaginal hypesthesis," there is orgasm in the clitoris but not the vagina, and, in the sixth, "frigidity of the nymphomaniac type," the woman feels "strong excitement, mounting repeatedly," but, of course, no vaginal orgasm.[63]

So fine, and at the same time, so arbitrary were these gradations, that it seems no simple matter to understand where any given woman belonged on the scale or just why it would be important to position her. The only thing that's clear is the overriding need to gather evidence about women's sexual responses, so that physicians could understand where they originated, their precise location and intensity, and could then talk about them in the most explicit terms. A couple of decades earlier, physicians had advised silence. As William Josephus Robinson wrote in *Married Life and Happiness* (1922): "Now, if you are one of those frigid or sexually anesthetic women, don't be in a hurry to inform your husband about it. To the man it makes no difference in the pleasurableness of the act whether you are frigid unless he knows that you are frigid. And he won't know unless you tell him, and what he doesn't know won't hurt him."[64] By contrast, mid-twentieth century physicians, particularly those with psychoanalytic training, were not merely interested in tracking down women's sexual sensations to their most hidden depths, they wanted to enroll their husbands in the enterprise.

With so much personal information at their disposal, psychiatrists and gynecologists, using the language and theoretical structures of Freudian psychoanalysis, not only managed to pass judgment on a woman's sexuality, they passed judgment on her marriage and family relations, and a host of other capacities and ways of functioning. To appreciate the reach of this discourse, to understand how frigidity came to inhabit and influence the most diverse pathologies, consider Hitschmann and Bergler's "Case A," an analysis of how sexual frigidity infiltrated and finally ruined every dimension of a twenty-six-year-old woman's life, making her "greedy, envious, hateful, sulky and vengeful," producing "general irritability," "evil temper toward the good-natured, self-sacrificing husband," inhibiting her "working capacity," while at the same time promoting "thoughts of killing her husband and marrying his brother" and "fantasies of murdering her child." And because frigidity implicated not only "Case A's" dreams, fantasies, and early childhood memories, but also the full range of her behavior in each of her adult relationships, curing her frigidity, according to Hitschmann–Bergler, produced a global transformation: "Through psychoanalysis she has changed into a happy being, capable of making others happy, glad of her motherhood, but also satisfying her ambition professionally. The vexatious, unhappy marriage, with the threat of adultery hanging over it, thus became permanently satisfying for both partners. A woman, freed from vaginal frigidity, has become a different and socially valuable person."[65]

To sum up, there was scarcely an attitude, feeling, or interpersonal event known to women from which mid-twentieth century Freudians could not impute some connection to frigidity. Not surprisingly, the vast majority of the attitudes, feelings, and behaviors associated with women's frigidity painted them in the darkest colors, particularly with regard to their affections for men. As Maurice Chideckel wrote in *Female Sex Perversion*, "frigid women, many of them, hate men. The hostile impulse toward the opposite sex becomes enhanced in many frigid women to such a degree that they would not stop at murder if they were not afraid of the consequences sure to follow."[66] According to Dr. Chideckel, the lovers and husbands of frigid women are naturally at greatest risk: "A woman unaware of her frigidity will admire a certain man for his manifold qualities, even permit him to kiss her. But soon after marriage she will belittle his merits, and actually hate him. She loved him until there was a demand for physical union. The thought of sexual contact causes a violent revulsion in her."[67]

The discourse that seemed obsessed with a woman's genitals, with their sensations and contractions, was also interested in her heart, her intentions, and her activities, with particular emphasis on the ways she performed as her husband's housekeeper and companion. As Marie Robinson formulated the discursive scope,

> the sad fact is that frigidity usually has a profound psychological connection on the individual. Her inadequacy is rooted in her childhood or adolescence, in early fears and misunderstandings, in events largely forgotten now. Around these early experiences, as crystals around a string, have clustered a whole series of personality traits that make life very hard for her and, much too often, unbearable for those nearest and dearest to her—her husband and her children.[68]

To illustrate the latter point, Robinson described how one of her frigid patients responded when she discovered her husband's pajamas on the bathroom floor and his shaving paraphernalia scattered around the sink. His messes "did not merely 'annoy' her; they 'enraged' her."[69] As far as Robinson's patient was concerned, they reflected her husband's desire to humiliate her, to demonstrate that she had nothing better to do than pick up after him and wait on him hand and foot. And the more the wife spoke on this, according to Robinson, the more hostile and belligerent she became, revealing how frigidity is not limited to sexual matters, nor is it best understood as a disease that only exists inside a woman.

Rather, frigidity affects every relationship she has and everything she does, in their totality.

Constructing Normal Women

As Bergler, Hitschmann, and other psychoanalytically trained physicians constructed the pathology and inferiority of the frigid, they simultaneously constructed the health and superiority of the non-frigid—"the startling antithesis between the frigid woman who responds with astonishment and coldness, even with disgust, envy and hate, to being kissed, touched or caressed, as well as to the sexual act itself, and the healthy woman who, warmly passionate and fully alive, accompanies the orgasm with cries of rapture."[70] To the degree physicians portrayed frigid neurotic women as unwilling to give men satisfaction in intercourse, to the degree they cited frigid women's disgust and revulsion ("When I have intercourse I feel like spitting. I can't stand my husband's hands on me. When I have to go to bed with him and there is no way out I feel trapped like an animal about to be slit open with a knife. I could strangle him and kick him"[71]), to that same degree they implicitly, and often explicitly, portrayed normal non-frigid women as delighted to give men the most satisfying intercourse experience imaginable. As gynecologist E. G. Hamilton explained in his article, "Frigidity in the Female" (1961), the normal, non-frigid woman

> is always ready to make love when her husband is ready (barring sickness, or certain times in pregnancy). Her deep altruism makes her extremely sensitive to his moods, and she will not find it in herself to treat him as if he were a robot, become angry or feel rejected if, when the button is pushed, he does not respond. She will die a thousand deaths rather than make him feel sexually inadequate.[72]

Hamilton went on to explain that a normal non-frigid woman always follows her husband's sexual lead. He decides whether they are going to make love, and the kind of lovemaking they will engage in, "and, in pure delight she follows him completely. Whether he feels lusty, gentle and tender, experimental or passive, she picks up the mood and responds delightedly."[73] From Frank Caprio's perspective, if it can be said that during the sex act, the frigid wife hears an inner voice telling her, "now is your time to display your sexual authority; push him, take the pleasure out of his affection," then, at the opposite pole, during the sexual act, the non-frigid wife hears an inner voice saying, "With my body I thee worship."[74]

To the degree that physicians characterized the sexually frigid in negative terms, to that same degree they characterized the non-frigid in positive terms, so that if a frigid wife "expresses her frustration in the form of nagging, irritability, temper tantrums, weeping spells, etc.,"[75] a non-frigid wife "must then be remorseless with herself and search for and exhume every last vestige of hostile and irrational emotion."[76] If the frigid wife always has "one complaint or other to lodge against her husband, humiliating him in company,"[77] the non-frigid wife, by contrast, recognizes that "her aggression is directed towards his enemies, never toward him."[78]

In other words, in this discourse, we always have the ideal of the normal non-frigid woman at the same time as—and precisely because—we have her antithesis. That the frigid woman is "full of anger and hatred for her husband" implies that the non-frigid woman listens, consoles, and helps him in any way she can,[79] and that her "watchwords are: Patience, tenderness, understanding and forgiveness."[80] That "frigid women are usually restrained, ill at ease and feel inadequate unless they are with their inferiors,"[81] that they are "easily angered, aggressive and jealous"[82] implies that the non-frigid woman "seeks agreement, unity, and her husband's happiness and peace of mind above all things. Having done this she has tapped the greatest psychologic joy of woman—that of giving."[83] In sum, frigidity discourse supported the ideals of female servility, sacrifice, selflessness, passivity, and denial, qualities that Marie Robinson collapsed into a single character trait called "essential female altruism," a virtue that reaches its fullest blossom in the ways a woman takes care of her children and husband: "She never resents this need in herself to give; she never interprets its manifestations as a burden to her, an imposition on her. It pervades her nature as the color green pervades the countryside in the spring, and she is proud of it and delights in it."[84]

If a frigid woman is incapable of seeing her husband for the man he truly is, if "his individual and essential quality is entirely unknown to her and unknowable to her,"[85] then, according to E. G. Hamilton, the non-frigid woman makes understanding her husband one of her most important duties: "By gaining such knowledge she is ultimately able to go to the very root of his personality, making an even deeper merging with him possible. Such understanding implies, of course, a great sensitivity to all his reactions. It makes her, too, inquire urgently (and creatively) into herself, so that no blocks to their deep psychologic communion can develop."[86]

The formula is consistent. Non-frigidity or normality in women equals giving to men; frigidity or abnormality equals withholding from men. A normal, non-frigid wife takes no respite from devotion. She lives in a continuous frenzy of selflessness and self-abasement before the needs of her husband and children. If she experiences any doubt—"any strange stirring"—she has to stop herself at the very threshold of that feeling and wipe it from consciousness.[87] According to Marie Robinson's *The Power of Sexual Surrender*, this repudiation is essential for four reasons. First, angry, rebellious feelings toward a husband are simply false: "They have no basis in fact; they do not pertain to the male *as he is*. . . . No matter how real these negative attitudes appear to be, remember that they are only feelings, not reality."[88] Second, the husband is an ally and protector:

> Far from seeking to enslave our sex, to exploit us through his strength and his aggression, man has put these two great and basic characteristics at our service. It is (and always has been) this fact that makes it safe for us to be women, to bear his children with a sense of security, to rear them knowing that he is there, always and forever, earning our bread, watching over us ceaselessly, keeping his terrible anxieties about us and our safety to himself so that we do not have to worry as he does.[89]

Third, the act of sexual surrender makes a woman beautiful: "Drawn expressions relax, anxious forehead wrinkles disappear, thin-lipped mouths soften. Indeed her whole body rounds and softens, taking on the look associated with a tender and giving femininity." Finally, sexual surrender produces fulfillment, a trance-like euphoria characterized by "a tremendous surging physical ecstasy in the feeling itself, in the feeling of being the passive instrument of another person, of being stretched out supinely beneath him, taken up will-lessly by his passion as leaves are swept up by the wind."[90]

The image of the normal non-frigid woman that emerges from these descriptions is much the same as the fluffy, passive feminine creature whom Betty Friedan described as "gaily content in the world of bedroom and kitchen, sex, babies, and home," the image that filled women's magazines such as *McCall's* and *Ladies Home Journal* during the 1950s.[91] Both portrayed women's subordinate role as natural, unalterable, and the source of innumerable advantages. The difference is that frigidity discourse came from physicians, and when physicians speak, people usually pay attention.

PART 2
BIRTH OF SEX THERAPY

3
Masters and Johnson and the Primacy of Intercourse

> The responsive, fully functioning man wants a responsive, fully functioning wife—a woman who has discovered her natural sexual capacity and who enjoys it.
> —Masters and Johnson, *The Pleasure Bond* (1970)

"Frigidity" was sanctioned as a diagnosis in the 1952 version of the *Diagnostic and Statistical Manual for Mental Disorders* (American Psychiatric Association) under the heading "Supplementary Terms of the Urogenital System," but did not appear in the 1968 version or any subsequent version. Between 1940 and 1979, the titles of 50 articles listed under *Psychological Abstracts* contained the word *frigidity* but none after 1979.[1] During the 1950s, every issue of *The Yearbook of Obstetrics & Gynecology* advised physicians to investigate patients for "true frigidity" following routine gynecological check-ups, but never again afterward.

The mid-twentieth century frigidity epidemic can be traced in part to the post-war idealization of marriage and large families, the growing belief that a woman's place is in the home,[2] and, of course, to the influence of Freud and psychoanalysis. Its fall can be traced to the rising influence of biological positivists such as Kinsey and Masters and Johnson and, perhaps most important, Masters and Johnson's texts, *Human Sexual Response* and *Human Sexual Inadequacy*.[3] While the authors claimed that the latter text offered "a *startlingly new approach* to the treatment of sexual problems,"[4] some have questioned that claim on the grounds that *Human Sexual Inadequacy* seemed to follow paths already well traversed by behaviorists such as Joseph Wolpe. Still, many others argued that Masters and Johnson deserve credit for the research that substantiated the theories and techniques of what was soon to become the sex therapy profession.[5] Helen Singer Kaplan explained:

> For two decades Masters and Johnson studied the sexual behavior of men and women under scientific laboratory conditions. They observed and recorded approximately 14,000 sexual acts. Their observations included a wide spectrum of sexual behavior under every imaginable condition. They studied coitus

in many positions, between strangers, between happily married couples, between couples who had various sexual and interpersonal difficulties. Different techniques of erotic stimulation were explored, as were various types of self-stimulation. . . . These studies finally yielded an accurate picture of the basic psychophysiology of human reproductive functioning. This information has had a tremendous impact on the field by opening up the possibility of the development of a rational and effective treatment of sexual disorders.[6]

Masters and Johnson introduced a level of rigor to sex therapy research that was completely foreign to their "frigidity" forebears, especially given the latter's reliance on case studies and anecdotal evidence, their disdain for controls and statistics, and their preoccupation with what can neither be observed nor measured—unconscious processes. As Masters and Johnson put it, the research methods that supported Freudian, psychoanalytic approaches to sex therapy were "derived more from the therapist's personal investment in the psychotherapeutic process than from an objective knowledge of sexual function or a practical application of behavioral principles."[7] According to Masters and Johnson, people who sought help from therapists steeped in the frigidity paradigm "were being treated with professional insight drawn either from the psychotherapist's own sexual experience—good, bad, or indifferent as it may have been—or from anecdotal material provided by previous patients."[8]

To fully understand why the "frigidity" paradigm fell from grace, we should also consider how much more cost-efficient the Masters and Johnson approach was. As Bergler himself acknowledged, treating a sexual dysfunction through Freudian, insight-oriented analysis did not make much sense for most people, since it required "an appointment several times a week for a minimum of eight months," which led him to conclude that "as a mass problem, the question of frigidity is unfortunately not to be solved."[9]

To add one more dynamic to the fall of "frigidity," we should consider the influence of second wave feminism. Beginning with Beard's critique of the "cult" of Freud,[10] by the late 1960s, feminist scholars had launched a full-scale assault on the Freudian practice of characterizing human traits as masculine or feminine,[11] with many focusing on the social and personal costs of marking women as sexually frigid. In Dana Densmore's words,

> the suffering that countless women have endured because they were told that if they didn't have vaginal orgasms they were frigid—that they were neurotic and selfish and unwomanly and sexually maladjusted and unable to let go and give and secretly resented the power of their husbands and envied them—this suffering is staggering and heartbreaking.[12]

Kinsey may have provided evidence that the center of sexual stimulation and orgasm for women is the clitoris and not the vagina more than a decade before Masters and Johnson,[13] but Masters and Johnson were the ones who succeeded in infiltrating the cultural imagination. They were the ones who got the idea across to the general public in articles published in magazines such as *Time* and *Newsweek*, always with somber portraits of themselves dressed in white lab coats.[14] They were scientific celebrities, and many women greeted their finding that the clitoris is the agent of women's orgasmic pleasure with a sense of vindication.[15] For feminists such as Anne Koedt, Masters and Johnson's research had a wonderfully liberating effect, since it not only debunked the myth of the vaginal orgasm; it also indicated "that sexual pleasure was obtainable from either men *or* women, thus making heterosexuality not an absolute, but an option. It would thus open up the whole question of *human* sexual relationships beyond the confines of the present male-female role system."[16] As William Masters assessed the sexual renaissance that he and Virginia Johnson had ushered in, "today the young woman is free to make her choice, pick her time, her place, her circumstance, without the old fears."[17] As Virginia Johnson characterized the new era, "the fact is that for the first time in many decades, the girl is running the sexual show. She is not a victim; she doesn't have to put up or shut up."[18]

These quotations are from a *Playboy* interview conducted in 1968 and suggest that Masters and Johnson's elevation to the status of feminist icons came with more than a few ironies. Among the most obvious is their failure to consider women's social disadvantages. As Ross Morrow observed in *Sex Research and Sex Therapy: A Sociological Analysis of Masters and Johnson* (2013), on the rare occasions when Masters and Johnson appeared to notice gender inequality, far from seeing it as something that should be factored into their treatment model, they dismissed it as a natural and, therefore healthy feature of social life.[19] They argued, for instance, that because a woman is naturally multiorgasmic,[20] because her "physiological capacity for sexual response infinitely surpasses that of man,"[21] it's only fair (and natural) that she should have some psycho-sexual-social disadvantages too. In Masters and Johnson's own words, "indeed, her significantly greater susceptibility to negatively based psychosocial influences may imply the existence of a natural state of psycho-sexual-social balance between the sexes that has been culturally established to neutralize women's biophysical superiority."[22]

Women's Liberation—On Men's Terms

Masters and Johnson not only appeared uninterested in the power differential between men and women, their sympathies seemed to rest with their male

52   BIRTH OF SEX THERAPY

patients. According to Janice Irvine in *Disorders of Desire: Sexuality and Desire in Modern American Sexology* (2005),[23] their pro-male bias was more than a sentimental preference—more than a simple matter of partiality—it was also a practical matter with the most tangible and far-reaching effects on the ways Masters and Johnson assessed and treated patients. Consider this case description from *Human Sexual Inadequacy*, from the chapter titled "Ejaculation Incompetence":

> The Jewish man was of orthodox belief. One night, at the age of 24 years, totally breaking with traditional behavior for the first and only time in his life, he not only forced physical attention upon, but tried to penetrate a young woman somewhat resistant to his approach. She stopped him with a plea that she was menstruating. He was devastated with this information, left her company as soon as physically possible, and never saw the woman again. As a result of this experience the subsequent two years were spent in psychotherapy.
>
> Four years later, this man married a young woman of similarly restrictive religious and social background. The courtship was severely chaste. In the marriage both husband and wife rigorously adhered to orthodox demands for celibacy within menstrual and postmenstrual time sequences. Every coital experience was potentially traumatic because, even with full erection and long-continued coital connection, the husband was unable to ejaculate intravaginally. His concept of the vagina as an unclean area had been reinforced by his traumatic premarital sexual experience. Such was his level of trauma that during marital coition, whenever the urge to ejaculate arose, the mental imagery of possible vaginal contamination drove him to withdraw immediately. A marriage of eight years had not been consummated when this marital unit was seen in therapy. During the two years before therapy, this man experienced an increasing number of instances of erectile failure with coital opportunity as his fears for sexual performance increased.[24]

What does Masters and Johnson's treatment of rape/attempted rape, as described here, say about their sensitivity to women's interests? In particular, consider their language, the way they described sexual assault. What does it mean to say that their patient "forced physical attention upon" and "tried to penetrate" a young woman? What does it mean that she was "somewhat resistant to his approach"? The answer is, We will never know, because Masters and Johnson either did not ask their patient or, if they did, felt the information too unimportant to share with readers.

What's behind these absences? Why didn't Masters and Johnson explore the details of that attack in the text, including the question of whether their patient's sexual dysfunction may have been caused, at least in part, by the fact that the woman who was menstruating was also his victim? Did their patient recognize that the woman he attacked was a person and not just a vagina? Did he understand and appreciate the concept of sexual consent? And, more generally, what role did sexual consent play in this man's marriage and in his value system? The problem here is that by failing to report on whether these questions were asked, Masters and Johnson not only rendered coercion invisible in their text; they positioned it as a normal part of men's and women's sexual relations. As Margaret Jackson summed up Masters and Johnson's record on this issue, "while they are usually careful to state that they do not condone sexual violence, they constantly trivialize its effects on women, or suggest that the women provoked it or even wanted and enjoyed it."[25]

Another example of Masters and Johnson's casual treatment of men's sexual domination of women, and, indeed, their casual treatment of the whole idea of gender inequality, appears in a very brief passage reporting how they treated a man suffering from what they called "secondary impotence." In this passage, they told how their patient, a man with a history of losing his erection during his attempts at vaginal penetration, "succeeded" one night in maintaining his erection long enough to accomplish penetration. However, Masters and Johnson offered few details on how he accomplished that penetration, and nothing on how the woman reacted. What should be noticed here, especially, is the complete absence of anything pertaining to the woman's consent.

> Three months after the initial episode of erective failure, he awoke with an erection, quickly mounted and ejaculated. His unprepared wife became pregnant.[26]

In this description, the woman appears briefly as a kind of background feature of her husband's sex life—an inanimate object whom he "mounted." Whatever he did to her, he did "quickly," when she was "unprepared," creating the impression that the wife may not have even been awake when her husband began to "mount" her. Other questions come to mind. Even if she had been awake, was she at all interested in having her husband insert his penis into her? Was she a willing partner? Or did she seem to resist in some way? Again, the absence of detail about her wakefulness, her desire, and her capacity to give sexual consent, and, perhaps most important, the absence of anything in the text pointing to Masters and Johnson's interest in obtaining these kinds of data, create the impression that, for Masters and Johnson, information of this type is not very important. For these therapists, the possibility that a man inserted his penis into the vagina of a sleeping woman does not appear to rank as a problem worth exploring. As a result of this apparent indifference, the vignette conveys the message that whether a man "mounts" his spouse when she is awake or sleeping, whether she desires sex or not, is not a primary concern. What matters more is that he has an opportunity to use his erection in the manner for which nature designed it—as an instrument of penetration.

That Masters and Johnson did not appear particularly invested in exploring the possibility of men's sexually coercive behavior suggests that they were also not particularly invested in exploring a range of other, less obvious forms of gender domination. To illustrate, consider Masters and Johnson's characterization of the way their clinic "helped" Mrs. B become a better, more satisfying sexual partner for her husband. According to the case description, the wife, who was fifty-seven years old at the time she began treatment at the Masters and Johnson clinic, had always been a reluctant sex partner. She claimed to find no pleasure in intercourse and only participated in sexual activity with her husband in response to his demands to fulfill her concept of a dutiful wife:

> She had never been orgasmic either during coition or with manipulation, nor had she ever attempted masturbation. She had always been sure that sexual function was only of interest to men, that "good" women never responded sexually, and that her only reward from sexual activity was reproduction.[27]

After she finally told her husband that she did not enjoy and did not want to continue having sex with him, he brought her to Masters and Johnson in what appears as an effort to change her attitude. At the clinic, her therapists attempted to reassure her that there was no reason why she couldn't continue to have sex with her husband into her sixties and beyond. But she was not reassured. In fact, "she was initially deeply disturbed, then quite angry, soon very distrustful and, at best, only minimally cooperative."[28] While "only minimally cooperative," she was, nonetheless, cooperative enough to consent to participate in the treatment program, which, as far as Masters and Johnson were concerned, turned out to be an unqualified success:

> Mrs. B became intrigued with the new information at her disposal, lost her high level of suspicion, grew totally cooperative, and in short order became fully responsive sexually. She actually was orgasmic during the acute phase of treatment.[29]

Masters and Johnson's version of this story may be entirely accurate. After Mrs. B had gone through their treatment program, she may have become orgasmic and "fully responsive sexually," exactly as Masters and Johnson claimed. However, an alternative, more complicated version of Mrs. B's story may also be true. In that version, we have a husband and wife who are at odds with regard to their sexual needs. He adamantly wants sex and she adamantly does not. To make her change her mind, he induces her to go to a sex therapy clinic where people are encouraged to have sex. She vigorously resists ("she was initially deeply disturbed, then quite angry"), but, after pressure from her husband and the Masters and Johnson staff, who side with him, she gives in. If we consider Robert Dahl's classic definition of power ("A has power over B to the extent that he can get B to do something that B would not otherwise do"[30]), then in the alternative version of what happened with this couple, the story is not about sex, but about power. This becomes a story of how the marital partner with less power, the wife, was induced or forced to acquiesce to the demands of the partner with more power, the husband. For Mrs. B, her husband's alliance with Masters and Johnson may have proven too formidable to oppose.

The main evidence supporting Masters and Johnson's version of events is Mrs. B's orgasms. They assumed that her sexual experience must have shifted from negative to positive because she was now having orgasms during intercourse. The problem here, of course, is that an orgasm is often experienced as involuntary and, furthermore, people are capable of having orgasms under the most disturbing, regrettable circumstances.[31] Consider, for example, that sometimes, in the midst of a sexual assault, the victim will experience physical sensations leading to orgasm,[32] which raises serious doubts about using orgasm, or a patient's claim of having an orgasm, as a sure-fire indicator of sexual enjoyment and satisfaction. This is especially true in light of the fact that victims of sexual assault sometimes fake orgasm as a means of bringing the assault to an end,[33] thus raising the question of whether B's reported orgasms really happened. In other words, it is possible that she felt compelled to fake orgasms as part of a strategy to disarm and appease her husband and therapists. She may have only said she had orgasms to quiet her inquisitors.

Obviously, we will never know the truth about Mrs. B's sexual responses—whether they occurred in the ways Masters and Johnson claimed, and if they did, what they really meant to her. We will never know if Mrs. B really felt that the Masters and Johnson treatment program helped her. All we know is that Masters and Johnson gave no indication of considering the role that gender inequality may have played in her story. All we know is that, in their text, Masters and Johnson gave no credence to Mrs. B's professed disinterest in sex, no credence to her angry plea to be left alone, and no credence to the possibility that sex therapy, far from enhancing Mrs. B's sexual autonomy, stifled its very emergence.

Intercourse *Ueber Alles*

Among the least publicized, and perhaps strangest, ironies associated with Masters and Johnson is their enthusiastic endorsement of heterosexual intercourse. One would imagine, much as Anne Koedt and other feminists have,[34] that their discovery of the clitoris' sexual power might have toppled penis–vagina intercourse, heterosexual men's preference, from its perch as the most accepted and obvious way of bringing women to orgasm. This might have been the moment when fingers, lips, tongue, and vibrator replaced the penis, or, at least, gained a place alongside the penis, as first-tier orgasmic options for women. But Masters and Johnson did not go down that path. Rather, in describing a woman's biologic readiness for heterosexual intercourse—how her vagina expands and lubricates in anticipation of a penis—Masters and Johnson made this sexual technique appear less like a sexual option for women than a mandate from nature:

> To appreciate vaginal anatomy and physiology is to comprehend the fundamentals of the human female's primary means of sexual expression. In essence, the vaginal barrel responds to effective sexual stimulation by involuntary preparation for penile penetration. Just as penile erection is a direct physiologic expression of a psychologic demand to mount, so expansion and lubrication of the vaginal barrel provides direct physiologic indication of an obvious psychologic mounting invitation. . . . The vagina truly provides a direct physiologic reflection of female psychosexual tensions, as it involuntarily prepares for and then accommodates the act of copulation.[35]

Consider that Masters and Johnson required their research subjects—those whom they used to establish baselines for normal sexual behavior—to have a "positive history" of reaching orgasm during intercourse.[36] The women Masters and Johnson studied to determine what normal sexuality is, had to have, as a condition of their employment, a proven "basic interest in and desire for effectiveness of sexual performance,"[37] coupled with a capacity to attain orgasm from a penis thrusting inside their vagina. Also consider that Masters and Johnson did not use the word *consummation* as a description of sex, except when referring to penis–vagina intercourse. As far as they were concerned, heterosexual couples could not *consummate* their marriage with fingers, lips, tongue, or vibrator; they could only *consummate* by means of a penis entering into a vagina, a physical act that did not have to be pleasurable to the woman or even consensual. For example, if we judge by Masters and Johnson's description of a couple's failed attempt at consummation, the failure was due, not to the woman patient's experience of pain or to the absence of consent; it failed because the overeager husband could not accomplish the physical act of penetration.[38]

> While attempting rapid consummation, his wife, unprepared for the physical onslaught, was hurt. She screamed; he lost his erection and could not regain function. By mutual agreement, further attempts at consummation were reserved for the seclusion of the wedding trip.[39]

How ironic that despite so much evidence of their women patients' discomfort with intercourse, Masters and Johnson continued to emphasize women's "natural" readiness for it. A central part of their endorsement of intercourse also involved de-emphasizing the many times and occasions that women (and men) are not ready for or interested in intercourse—the many times and occasions intercourse is unrewarding and ill-advised, not to mention profoundly disturbing, even lethal, given its association with violence, unwanted conception, and sexually transmitted diseases. Instead, Masters and Johnson portrayed penis–vagina intercourse as a kind of biological gift, indispensable to a woman's, as well as a man's, well-being and pleasure:

> The functional role of a penis is that of providing an organic means for physiologic and psychologic increment and release of *both male and female sexual tensions*.[40]

Their assumption of the goodness and naturalness of intercourse for both men and women appears so deeply entwined in their research and therapy that, at times, they simply take its probity for granted, as illustrated by how easily they appeared to slide, without transition, from descriptions of the physiology of a woman's orgasm to descriptions of her physiology during intercourse (coitus), almost as if, in their minds, orgasm and coitus are interchangeable:

> At orgasm, the grimace and contortion of a woman's face graphically express the increment of myotonic tension throughout her entire body. The muscles of the neck and the long muscles of the arms and legs usually contract into involuntary spasm. During coition in supine position the female's hands and feet voluntarily may be grasping her sexual partner.[41]

In their very next sentence, Masters and Johnson introduced "automanipulative techniques"—their term for masturbation—as another way to bring women to orgasm.[42] Indeed, they routinely encouraged the women in their treatment program to masturbate and to share masturbation techniques. But as Janice Irvine pointed out in *Disorders of Desire*, Masters and Johnson's discussion of masturbation mainly focused on how it can be used as a means of staying in shape for and learning about intercourse.[43] In other words, Masters and Johnson encouraged women who have had difficulty reaching orgasm in intercourse to masturbate, not as an end in itself, but as a tool for learning how to achieve successful orgasm in intercourse. While Masters and Johnson devoted a great deal of attention to formulating and describing the pleasures of sensual touching and masturbation, they seemed to always treat touching and masturbation as distant runners-up to intercourse, as evidenced by the following vignette, where masturbation appears as a somewhat embarrassing way for a woman to "resolve her own sexual tensions" at a time when she believes she has lost her husband as a viable intercourse partner:

> Their sexual dysfunction had begun when the husband was 57 year old. He had noted some delay in attaining erection and marked reduction in ejaculatory volume and was particularly concerned with the fact that the ejaculatory experience was one of a mere dribbling of seminal fluid from the external urethral meatus, under obviously reduced pressure. All these involutional signs and symptoms developed within approximately a year after he had noticed some delay in onset of erection attainment. The more he worried about his symptoms the more frequent the occasions of impotence.
>
> Mrs. B was completely convinced that this pattern was indeed to be expected as part of the aging process. Rather than distress her husband, she suggested they use separate bedrooms. She changed from a pattern of free and easy exchange of sexual demand to one of availability of coital connection only at her husband's expression of interest. In order to resolve her own sexual tensions, she masturbated about once every ten days to two weeks without her husband's knowledge.[44]

For Masters and Johnson, masturbation appears as a method for surviving during sexual dry spells, when access to heterosexual partners is limited or unavailable.[45] Rather than go through long periods of stressful sexual abstinence, which might lead to the atrophy of sexual organs and reflexes, they advanced masturbation as an effective way for people without partners to maintain their equanimity and readiness for what matters most—intercourse. This prioritization of intercourse is nowhere more apparent than in the ways they defined individuals' sexual dysfunctions. Accordingly, for Masters and Johnson, a man's main sexual dysfunction is either his inability to attain an erection rigid enough to penetrate a vagina or, once inside, his inability to ejaculate at the appropriate time, with the appropriate volume and intensity. Similarly, a woman's main sexual dysfunction is either her inability to accept a penis into her vagina or, once she has accepted it, her inability to have an orgasm in response to penile thrusting.[46]

The prioritization of intercourse is also apparent in how Masters and Johnson described therapy aimed at helping individuals overcome their sexual dysfunctions. For the man who cannot ejaculate, for example—"the incompetent ejaculator"—the first step in therapy is for "the wife to force ejaculation manually," although ejaculation, in and of itself, is not the final goal. The final goal always involves a penis inside a vagina. "After establishing competence in ejaculatory function with masturbatory techniques, the next step toward intravaginal ejaculatory response is in order."[47] In this step, the wife is supposed to stimulate her husband with her hands until he reaches "ejaculatory inevitability." She then attempts to rapidly insert his penis into her vagina: "Once the coital connection is established, a demanding style of female pelvic thrusting against the captive penis should be instituted immediately. Usually this teasing technique is sufficient to accomplish ejaculation shortly after intromission."[48]

For men who have difficulty getting an erection, the first step in their therapeutic exercises, again, is "manipulative play," followed by an interval of quiet, and "then return to play and resurgence of erective attainment."[49] Once the man's erection recurs through his wife's manual assistance, she is supposed to insert his penis into her vagina: "When or if full erection is obtained, the wife may mount, but intromission should be attempted in a nondemanding manner. No hurry to mount—no rush to obtain sexual tension release—should be permitted."[50] Intercourse should proceed slowly and calmly, in a nondemanding manner, because "impotent men having achieved intromission successfully still have not satisfied their performance fears. They immediately question whether the penis will retain sufficient rigidity for continuation of coition."[51]

Once men are confident that their penis will remain rigid long enough to continue coition, they have one more obstacle to overcome. "They immediately question whether the penis will retain sufficient rigidity for continuation of effective coital connection,"[52] which raises the question: What did Masters and Johnson mean by "effective coital connection?" The answer: A coital connection that lasts long enough to "satisfy" a woman.

> On occasion, 30 to 60 seconds of intravaginal containment is quite sufficient to satisfy a woman, if she has been highly excited during precoital sex play and is fully ready for orgasmic release with the initial thrusts of the penis. However, during most coital opportunity, the same woman may require variably longer periods of penile containment before attaining full release of sexual tension.
>
> While readily admitting the inadequacies of the definition, the Foundation [Masters and Johnson's Reproductive Biology Research Foundation] considers a man a premature ejaculator if he cannot control his ejaculatory process for a sufficient length of time during intravaginal containment to satisfy his partner in at least 50 percent of their coital connections.[53]

Masters and Johnson believed that the longer a man continues thrusting his penis inside a woman's vagina, the greater the likelihood that she will have an orgasm, although, oftentimes, things don't go as planned: "The husband fears that he will not be able to sustain an erection quality sufficient to satisfy his sexual partner."[54] Why should a husband have this sort of fear? Once again, it's because, for Masters and Johnson, a penis thrusting inside a woman's vagina is not only the most natural way for her to reach orgasm; it's the measure of a man's sexual success. While other sexual discourses may have claimed that "nature intended" men to give women babies, in Masters and Johnson's discourse, nature intended men to give women orgasms. And a man who fails in this mission—a man who, during intercourse, cannot maintain his erection long enough to bring his female partner to climax, warrants one of several possible stigmata, such as "premature ejaculator," "incompetent ejaculator," "a man with primary impotence," "a man with secondary impotence," or "a man with secondary impotence with homosexuality as contributing etiological factor."

For their female patients, Masters and Johnson promulgated complementary mythologies, along with complementary exercises. Thus, a woman who cannot achieve orgasm through intercourse is labeled "a nonorgasmic woman." According to Masters and Johnson, a woman so afflicted needs to remove the fears and negative attitudes that are interfering with her receptivity to her partner's sexual approach. And the way to do it, the way to remove those fears and blockages, is conceptually no different from the way they are removed in a man's treatment: she has to engage in a series of sexual exercises that may begin with manual foreplay and genital stimulation, but always have the same end-point—coition:

> Subsequent to reported success in manual genital excitation, the marital partners are asked to try the female-superior coitus position, by which means the wife may translate previously established levels of sensate pleasure into an experience which includes the sensation of penile containment.[55]

Even when a woman has a history of experiencing spasms or pain during intercourse, the goal appears the same: to have her accept a penis into her vagina, followed by her orgasm. To illustrate, in the following vignette involving a newly married twenty-six-year-old woman, Masters and Johnson drew the path, clearly and directly, from problem to cure, the problem being the woman's inability to allow penetration and the cure being her new-found ability to do so. They made this clear and direct link by failing to entertain the possibility that she might not want a penis in her vagina. Instead, they simply assumed the rightness of that proposition:

> Sexual exposure during the [couple's] short engagement had been restricted, by female edict, to multiple manipulative approaches. There was total inability to penetrate on the wedding night or to consummate the marriage thereafter. When the unit [the couple] was seen after 18 months of marriage, the wife's hymen was not intact but there was evidence of severe vaginismus.
> Once all of her pertinent history was obtained and shared with her marital partner, *there was little further resistance to penile penetration*. She was orgasmic

with intercourse within two weeks after termination of the acute phase of treatment.[56]

The most interesting feature of this very brief vignette is Masters and Johnson's evidence of treatment success, the relative absence of "resistance to penile penetration." This is worth thinking about, as are several related questions: What was the nature of this woman's original resistance? How did Masters and Johnson define "little further resistance to penile penetration?" And why did Masters and Johnson gloss over the man's attempt to get his penis into the vagina of a woman who was showing signs of resistance? How did he finally manage to get his penis into her vagina? Did he go against her wishes, violate her consent? Most important, why didn't Masters and Johnson provide a record of whether the woman was consulted on the nature and meaning of her resistance? Why was her testimony excluded from the case study? Finally, why are there no anecdotes in Masters and Johnson's text of male patients who are required to perform (undergo) sex acts despite their resistance? Why does *Human Sexual Inadequacy* only contain anecdotes of women who, as part of their treatment, are pressed to copulate against their will?

Because Masters and Johnson did not provide answers to these questions—indeed, did not even formulate these questions—in their account, a woman's resistance to intercourse does not appear to be a matter of great consequence to them. What matters more is the accomplishment of intercourse. Apparently, for Masters and Johnson, penetration—assertive, even forceful penetration—is an acceptable method of treating a woman's alleged intercourse failure.

If a woman's sexual dysfunction—vaginismus—is defined as her inability to accept a penis into her vagina, then curing that dysfunction requires the undoing of that inability. Following that logic, pressing her to accept a penis into her vagina is warranted on the grounds that it might cure her sexual dysfunction. This probably explains why the other vaginismus cases cited by Masters and Johnson reveal the same pattern. In none was the woman diagnosed with vaginismus comfortable imagining a penis entering her vagina. Indeed, most vaginismus sufferers described the idea as frightening and repulsive. Yet for all, intercourse was treated as necessary, sometimes as a method as well as a goal. Masters and Johnson appeared to tacitly assume that a woman who resists accepting a penis into her vagina has to overcome that deficiency if treatment is to succeed:

> Marital Unit D [couple D] was seen with the complaint of increasing difficulty in accomplishing vaginal penetration developing after 6 years of marriage. There were two children in the marriage, with onset of severe dyspareunia oriented specifically to the delivery of the second child. The second child, a post

mature baby of 8 pounds and 14 ounces, had a precipitous delivery. There was a positive history of nurses' holding the patient's legs together to postpone delivery while waiting for the obstetrician. As soon as sexual activity was reconstituted after the delivery the patient experienced severe pain with deep penile thrusting. During the next year the pain became so acute that the wife sought subterfuge to avoid sexual exposure. The coital frequency decreased from two to three times a week to the same level per month. On numerous occasions the patient was assured, during medical consultation, that there was nothing anatomically disoriented in the pelvis and that pain with intercourse was "purely her imagination."

Supported by these authoritative statements, the husband demanded increased frequency of sexual function. When the wife refused, the unit separated for 10 months. During this 10-month period, the woman assayed intercourse on two separate occasions with two different men, but with each experience the pelvic pain with deep penile thrusting was so severe that her obvious physical distress terminated sexual experimentation.

The marital unit was reunited with the help of their religious advisor, but with attempted intercourse vaginal penetration was impossible. After 8 months of repeatedly unsuccessful attempts to reestablish coital function, the unit was referred for therapy.[57]

Masters and Johnson did not document Mrs. D's desire to have a penis in her vagina, if indeed she ever had such a desire. Nor did they attempt to document their need, or any other therapist's need, to obtain this kind of information. Yet, according to their text, they proceeded with Mrs. D's cure, attempting to force a penis into her vagina, as they appeared to do in all other cases involving a woman who showed any difficulty accepting intercourse, with an unwavering faith that copulation is the natural end-point of human sexuality. This passage is illuminating:

If the female partner complains and flinches at penile insertion, moans and contracts her abdominal and pelvic musculature during the continuum of male thrusting, cries out or screams with deep vaginal penetration, sheds bitter tears after termination of every sexual connection, or complains angrily of aching in the pelvis or burning in the vagina during or even after a specific coital episode, the male partner's sexual approach must be accepted as the probable potentiator of a physiological basis for his female partner's evidenced sexual dysfunction. Thereafter the husband has minimal recourse. There is little he can do other than to avoid or at least reduce marital-unit sexual exposure on his own cognizance, and/or to insist that his wife seek professional consultation.[58]

For Masters and Johnson, according to their depictions of how they treat women with vaginismus, a woman may moan and cry out from the pain of intercourse, she may display all the signs of agony, but this does not necessarily mean her partner should cease his efforts. Rather, it means that he, not she, faces an enormous challenge, and with very limited options. He, not she, has some tough choices to make—whether to "avoid or at least reduce marital-unit sexual exposure on his own cognizance, and/or insist that his wife seek professional consultation."

Masters and Johnson did not appear to consider the choices that the woman, the one who is suffering from intercourse, has to make. They focused instead on the choices available to the man, the person whose pleasure might be interrupted. Thus, Masters and Johnson did not imagine the husband, or anyone else, asking the wife if she wants to seek professional consultation; rather, the husband's choice, as they saw it, was to "insist" that she go. What does this mean? In saying that a husband should "insist" that his wife receive treatment for her copulative inadequacy, were Masters and Johnson suggesting that she's incompetent? Did they believe, on some level, that she's the sexual property of her husband? Whatever the answer, it is hard to avoid the conclusion that Masters and Johnson did not believe that Mrs. D., or any other woman who resists intercourse because of pain, or any other reason, should be supported in her resistance.

Apparently, for Masters and Johnson, the necessity of intercourse was not a falsifiable proposition. Instead, it functioned much like the law of inertia or the indestructibility of matter, as an incorrigible principle. A woman's distress at the prospect or experience of intercourse, in fact, a whole lifetime of such distress, did not alter their conviction that this sex act has been encoded by nature as *the* way to consummate marriage.

For them, penis–vagina intercourse superseded all other sexual activities. Despite their finding that a woman's orgasm affects her entire body, producing especially intense feelings in her clitoris, they continued to emphasize penis–vagina intercourse over the direct and separate manipulation of the clitoris, as the shortest, most precise route to a woman's sexual pleasure and orgasm. They defended this bias on the grounds that the clitoris "is an extremely tender area, which the female rarely manipulates herself. She more or less stimulates herself along the shaft or just in the general clitoral area, which is called the mons."[59] Here is how William Masters explained that the man's thrusting during heterosexual intercourse, while avoiding direct contact with the highly sensitive clitoris glans, brings just enough contact onto the shaft of the clitoris to bring a woman to orgasm:

> The clitoris is stimulated during intercourse every time the female responds to the male thrust. The reaction occurs regardless of what position she may be in.

You see, with each thrust, the minor labia are pulled down toward the rectum and, in the process, stimulate the shaft of the clitoris.[60]

No matter that Masters and Johnson arrived at this conclusion by only studying women who are able to attain orgasm through intercourse and that the minor labia are only pulled down in this manner, producing traction with the clitoris, when a woman is already in a high state of arousal.[61] No matter that most women say they cannot reach orgasm from penis–vagina intercourse, many say they have no desire for it, and many others say they cannot tolerate it.[62] For Masters and Johnson, penis–vagina intercourse occupies a special status, as a sexual activity designed by nature for a woman's anatomy.[63]

Freudians versus Masters and Johnson

Why, then, do women often fail to attain orgasm during heterosexual intercourse? Masters and Johnson's answer to this question is ironic, especially in view of their much publicized disdain for psychoanalysis and its approaches to sexual frigidity. For them, as for Freud and his followers, a woman fails to reach orgasm during sexual intercourse, not because she finds this activity inherently unrewarding or unpleasurable. It's because something is interfering with her inborn capacity to appreciate intercourse and attain vaginal orgasm. As previously mentioned, Freud likened an individual's sexual inhibition to "a stream whose main bed has been blocked." Thus, for Freud, Dora's problem was not that she found Herr K.'s sexual advances repulsive; her problem was that some kind of fear was blocking her "natural" attraction to him. So too for Masters and Johnson, the problem is not that some women, or some men, have an inherent distaste for, or disinterest in, broccoli; the problem is that some kind of fear is blocking their hard-wired love for broccoli. They describe sexual inhibition as originating in "fear in all its forms: the fear of being hurt, physically or emotionally; the fear of being wrong or making a mistake and being punished or ridiculed; the fear of being considered ugly, clumsy, foolish, incompetent, unresponsive, undesirable . . . an almost endless list that includes every negative thought that human beings have ever had about themselves."[64]

This may explain why Masters and Johnsons used the word "natural" repeatedly, perhaps more than any other adjective, to communicate their belief that, despite people's complaints that they don't feel sexual desire, arousal, or orgasm, those capacities are inborn, already present, just waiting to be released:

> An original and continuing premise of our treatment model is that sexual response is natural. . . . Just as the natural physiological functions of respiration,

digestion, and urination are not taught to the newborn infant, the reflex pathways of sexual response cannot be taught.[65]

As Marny Hall (2001) described her experience at the Masters and Johnson sex therapy program at UCLA in her article, "Not Tonight Dear, I'm Deconstructing a Headache":

> We were taught that sex was a natural function—a set of responses so universal that it obliterated differences in sexual orientation, and even gender. Our instructors assured us that if the blocks to eroticism—ignorance, prudery, and performance anxiety—were removed, Mother Nature would reassert herself with vigor, whether our clients were gay or straight, men or women.[66]

My point is that the Freudian and Masters–Johnson treatment approaches share the belief that a therapist does not need to, and, indeed, cannot, implant or teach sexual desire. As Masters and Johnson put it, "This is like believing that we can be taught how to sweat or to make our hearts beat."[67] For Masters and Johnson, the idea of implanting sexual desire is absurd; it's absurd because sexual desire is already there, regardless of the patient's claims to the contrary. The problem—the reason for the individual's sexual dysfunction—is that the individual has learned to deny, divert, repress, or suppress those naturally occurring sexual energies. She has learned to sabotage her natural sexuality. As Masters and Johnson explained,

> many individuals seek counseling on the assumption that there are reliable methods of teaching sexual response. This is not quite accurate. What does exist is the possibility of identifying the obstacles to effective sexual functioning and that have removed sex from its natural context and suggesting ways to alleviate and/or circumvent those obstacles.... When this is done, natural function usually takes over with surprising ease.[68]

In other words, both the Freudian and the Masters and Johnson approaches assume that the treatment of sexual dysfunctions requires the removal, elimination, reconstruction, and/or diversion of the obstacles to normal sexual functioning. Moreover, they share the belief that what makes an obstacle to sexual functioning effective—what gives it the power to block an individual's naturally occurring sexual energy—is its capacity to generate fear and anxiety.

While Masters and Johnson dispelled the Freudian myth of the superiority of the vaginal orgasm and the inferiority of the clitoris, what is hardly ever acknowledged is their debt to Freud—how much of their understanding and treatment of sexual dysfunction is modelled on Freudian theory. Certainly,

Masters and Johnson and the Freudians had many differences. Masters and Johnson only treated couples, and always with two therapists. The treatment they offered at their clinic was briefer and more intense, with daily sessions lasting two or three weeks. They didn't assume that sexual dysfunction implied some kind of underlying psychopathology. Their treatment was also much more scripted. No self-respecting Freudian would ever begin treatment with a predetermined list of questions on sexual intercourse, as Masters and Johnson did: "How frequently do you recall having intercourse during the first month of your marriage? The first year of marriage? Did you enjoy this frequency?" "What has had the most influence on when or how often or under what circumstances you and your (husband, wife) have intercourse?" "Does lovemaking always lead to intercourse? If not, give percentage estimate." "Does coital activity usually grow out of shared moments of mutual emotional understanding, or is it scheduled?" "Does coition seem to occur from habit or a sense of duty?" "Do you have a preference for a particular time of day and situation for lovemaking?" "Do you feel the need to be physically close or to be held after intercourse? Does your partner express a similar need?" "Do you summon particular images or fantasies during intercourse? If so, describe." "In what kinds of petting (making out) did you participate ... [that progressed] to intercourse. If so, describe the first occasion. If so, what means of contraception was used (if any)?" "Under what circumstances did intercourse usually occur? How much pleasure and freedom from concern accompanied the experience? Were you ever suspected or caught? Punished?"[69]

But Masters and Johnson had many other, much broader, questions in their script. Like the Freudians, they wanted to know about their patients' personal development and background: how they functioned in their marriages, the psychic traumas they may have endured, their prior experiences with counseling and religious training, and the ways their symptoms developed and were shaped by their parental and other family relationships. Thus, in treating Mrs. A, Masters and Johnson paid particular attention to how her sexual problem—an inability to "consummate" her marriage—had its genesis in her family of origin: how, instead of being taught that sex is a natural and necessary part of life, she was taught that sex, in all its manifestations, is wrong:

> The young woman described a cold, formal, controlled family environment in which there was complete demand for dress as well as toilet privacy. Not only were the elder brother and sisters socially isolated, but the sisters also were given separate rooms and encouraged to protect individual privacy. She never remembers having seen her mother, father, brother, or sister in an undressed state. The subject of sex was never mentioned, and all literature, including newspapers, available to the family group was evaluated by her father

for possibly suggestive or controversial material. There was a restricted list of radio programs to which the children could listen.[70]

For Masters and Johnson, like the Freudians, the first step to overcoming the sexual negativity inherited from childhood is to obtain a psychological history. Talking about the problem's genesis, and relating it to the individual's present functioning, to some degree, neutralizes the problem. Where Masters and Johnson differed most radically from the Freudians was in the second step, which consisted of the direct dissemination of information. If Mrs. A, through daily exposure to her family's values, came to see sexuality as dirty, sinful, shameful, unpredictable, bizarre, frightening, and painful, then the solution, according to Masters and Johnson, is to tell her the truth about sex: tell her it's natural. Instead of inciting Mrs. A to speak about her sexual experiences and fantasies ad infinitum, instead of commanding her, as a psychoanalyst might have done, to transform her every desire into discourse, she, like other women attending the Masters and Johnson treatment program, was encouraged to listen and learn. She, like other women, had to be taught the science of sex:

> Women handicapped sexually by the influence of religious orthodoxy, married to men with sexual dysfunction, victimized by rape, contending with unexplained dyspareunia, frustrated by aging constriction of the vaginal barrel, or confused by homosexual and heterosexual conflict all have one thing in common. They all exhibit almost complete lack of authoritative information from which to gain some degree of objectivity when facing the psychosocial problem evidenced by the symptoms of their sexual dysfunction.
>
> With no knowledge of what to expect sexually, no concept of natural levels of sexual responsivity, and even real distrust for authority, theirs is a desperate need for definitive information.[71]

A Sensory Subject

Masters and Johnson also differed from the Freudians on the desirability of incorporating structured exercises into therapy that are designed to counteract and erase years of negative sexual conditioning. Thus, Masters and Johnson asked women who had been raised to believe that sex is shameful and wrong, or who had been sexually traumatized, either through rape or some other kind of assault, to participate in a reconditioning program that would help them experience sex as safe, gentle, non-threatening, and non-demanding. For example, for their first homework assignment at the Masters and Johnson clinic, couples were typically assigned "sensate focus" exercises that involved nothing more and nothing less than giving and receiving pleasure. In these exercises, couples were asked to focus completely on the physical sensations they could provide each other, on the ways they could touch and caress, without any conversation pertaining to each other's personality, history, or future, or any thoughts of achieving orgasm or any other outcome or performance goal. All that matters in these exercises, as well as in Masters and Johnson's other sexual exercises, is the sensory moment. This is how sensate focus instructions are worded:

> I'd like you both to get ready for bed—to take your clothes off, shower, and relax. I want you [the woman] to lie on your belly. Then you [the man] caress her back as gently and sensitively as you can. Move your hands very slowly. Begin at the back of her neck, caress her ears, and work your way down to her buttocks, legs, and feet. Use your hands and/or your lips. Concentrate only on how it feels to touch her body and her skin.
>
> In the meantime, I want you [the woman] to focus your attention on the sensations you feel when he caresses you. Try not to let your mind wander. Don't think about anything else, don't worry about whether he's getting tired, or whether he is enjoying it—or anything. Be 'selfish,' and just concentrate on your sensations; let yourself feel everything. Communicate with him. Don't talk too much or it will interfere with your responses—and his. But remember that he can't possibly know what you are feeling unless you tell him. Let him know where you want to be touched and how, and where his caresses feel especially good; and let him know if his touch is too light or too heavy, or if he is going too fast. If the experience is unpleasant, tell him so. Try to identify those areas of your body which are especially sensitive or responsive.
>
> When you have both had enough of this, I want you [the woman] to turn over on your back, so that you [the man] can caress the front of her body. Start with her face and neck and go down to her toes. But this time don't caress her sexual organs. Skip her nipples, her vagina and clitoris. Again, both of you can concentrate only on what it feels like to caress and be caressed. Stop when this becomes tedious for either of you. Now it's your [the man's] turn to receive. I want you [the woman] to do the same to him. Do either of you have any questions about this procedure.[72]

Perhaps the simplest, and most influential, feature of sensate focus exercises consists of asking couples to avoid goal-oriented sexual activity, a feature that characterizes almost all Masters and Johnson's exercises. Thus, on day one of sex therapy at the Masters and Johnson clinic, couples were "requested to refrain from overt sexual activity until otherwise directed."[73] Intercourse and orgasm were prohibited. What's behind this directive, according to Masters and Johnson, is the conviction that the main obstacle to successful sexual functioning is the culturally imposed pressure to achieve sexual success:

> The popular magazines, with their constant consideration of the subject, have brought to the nonorgasmic female a realization that in truth she is a naturally functional sexual entity. Unfortunately they have also provided her with real fears of performance by depicting, often with questionable realism, the sexual goals of effectively responsive women. Her frequently verbalized anxieties when she does not respond to the level of orgasm (at least a certain percentage of the time) are: "What is wrong with me?" "Am I less than a woman?" "I certainly must be physically unappealing to my husband," and so on. These grave self-doubts and usually groundless suspicions are translated into fear of performance.[74]

As Masters and Johnson conceptualized this problem, the more sexual partners fear performance failure, the more they sacrifice spontaneity. With increased fear and self-consciousness, sex becomes less about sharing feelings and more about conforming to sexual stereotypes and conventions. The tragic consequence of "performance fear" and "the spectator role," according to Masters and Johnson, is that sexual performers begin to feel and act robotic. They become desensitized—impervious to sexual stimuli; they are more likely to feel that they are only going through the motions, thus confirming their own worst fears: that they really are slow to respond, really are not very good at sex, and really aren't very attractive. Masters and Johnson called performance fear *"the greatest known deterrent to effective sexual functioning, simply because it so completely distracts the fearful individual from his or her natural responsivity by blocking reception of sexual stimuli either created by or reflected from the sexual partner."*[75]

Masters and Johnson got the idea of "performance fear" as an obstacle to successful sexual performance from an eighteenth century text, *Treatise on Venereal Disease*. The author, an English physician named John Hunter, theorized that for an individual to perform intercourse well, "the mind should be in a state entirely disengaged from everything else; it should have no difficulties, no fears, no apprehensions; not even an anxiety to perform the act well."[76]

Masters and Johnson's main contribution to Hunter's theory was to expand its scope to include couples. For example, at some point, the husband of a nonorgasmic woman may begin worrying about his wife's reaction to his erection or to the timing of his ejaculation: "He worries about why he, as a sexually functional man, cannot give her the 'gift' of response. Why is his wife nonresponsive to his sexual approaches? What really is wrong when he cannot satisfy her sexual needs?"[77] Masters and Johnson argued that a wife's inability to have an orgasm might make her husband more self-conscious, more on the spot to achieve performance success, and this added pressure might interfere with his capacity to respond to her spontaneously and naturally. He might then blame his wife, and she, as she becomes aware of his hostility, might blame herself (or him), which might, in turn, make her feel all the more inhibited.

While Masters and Johnson showed that the interactive effects of performance fear are virtually endless, they also expanded the scope of the treatment techniques available for addressing these dysfunctions. Instead of recommending, simply, that people take a break from intercourse, as Hunter did, Masters and Johnson separated, analyzed, and differentiated each sexual dysfunction down to its component parts. As a result, they not only came up with specific recommendations for how people should take breaks from intercourse, they came up with ideas on what should be done during breaks, how much time should elapse between intervals, and the steps required to resume normal sexual functioning—how each action should be measured, sustained, and finally superseded by the next logical advance. For example, for the "squeeze technique," designed to delay ejaculation, they calculated the time required for each squeeze, how much pressure the wife should apply to her husband's penis, the fingers she should use, and how her fingers should be positioned:

> Pressure is applied by squeezing the thumb and first two fingers together for an elapsed time of 3 to 4 seconds. If the man is uncircumcised, the coronal ridge still can be palpated and the first and second fingers correctly positioned. An approximation of frenulum positioning must be estimated for thumb placement.[78]

Similarly, for the woman suffering from orgasmic dysfunction, Masters and Johnson hypothesized that rehabilitation is not simply a matter of telling her to hold off and not worry about orgasm for a period of time, it is about partitioning her movements and sensations, breaking them down into their smallest parts, and then telling her what she should think of them, what attitudes and feelings she should have. For Masters and Johnson, no sensory or physiological detail appeared too unimportant, too fussy. Thus, the woman who has difficulty achieving orgasm is not only instructed how to move her body, but how she should react to her own movements, how she should interpret her own sensations and respond to them.

> When the marital partners extend their psychosensory interchange to coition in the female-superior position, the wife once mounted is instructed to hold herself quite still and simply to absorb the awareness of penile containment. Interspersed with moments of sensate pleasure created by her proprioceptive awareness of vaginal dilation should be the opportunity to feel and think

sexually. The vaginal distention should be interpreted in relation to the sensual desire for further increment in sexual pleasure. This increasing demand for sexual stimulation can be further implemented by the female partner if she will institute a brief period of controlled, slowly exploring, pelvic thrusting. The husband's specific responsibility at this moment is to provide the needed erect penis without any concept of a demanding thrusting pattern on his part. In anticipation of her need, the cotherapists must encourage the wife to think of the encompassed penis as hers to play with, to feel, and to enjoy, until the urge for more severe pelvic thrusting involuntarily emerges into her levels of conscious demand.[79]

The most interesting feature of these instructions is what they leave out. What is missing is the matter of whether the woman "once mounted" in the "female-superior position" actually wants to "absorb the awareness of penile containment." How much do women care about the "moments of sensate pleasure created by [their] proprioceptive awareness of vaginal dilation?" What, if anything, do they get out of the "brief period of controlled, slowly exploring, pelvic thrusting" performed with "the needed erect penis" inside their vagina? Does a woman really want "to think of the encompassed penis" as a standalone body part? Does she really want to think of it "as hers to play with, to feel, and to enjoy," as if it were some kind of sex toy?

Of course, women are different. There is no single, generic sexual model that covers all women. At the same time, researchers have consistently found that women are less likely than men to link their sexual satisfaction to the mechanics of intercourse and orgasm.[80] As Rosalind Gill and Rebecca Walker explain in their article, "Heterosexuality, Feminism, Contradiction: On Being Young, White, Heterosexual Feminists in the 1990s,"

> it is not just that penetration can feel like one more invasion, or simply that we find it less pleasurable than other forms of sexual contact, or only that it has always held particular dangers for women—and never more so than today. It is all these things, but it is also that it feels such an impoverished view of [our] sexual potential.[81]

After Shere Hite, in her groundbreaking study of women's sexuality, asked women to describe what they get and don't get out of sex, she discovered that their primary interest is not physical stimulation, sensory pleasure, and/or relief from sexual tension, but rather, emotional connection with a partner. Hite found that the fundamental reference point of a woman's sexual experience is not the body and its sensations, as Masters and Johnson emphasized. It's the person who inhabits the body. It's her relationship with her partner. What matters most to her is not the thrusting of a penis inside her vagina, so much as the infinite variety of ways thrusting and other sexual movements can be understood as indicators of intention and affection. For many women, sex isn't only a physical thing, and it's definitely not a rigid pattern of penetration followed by mutual orgasm. Rather, it's a flexible, mutual kind of communication—a sharing—freely chosen and non-coercive, tailored to each partner's needs, and centered on love and closeness.[82]

All of which suggests that Masters and Johnson's most significant omission may have been their failure to take into consideration the variety of ways women seek and respond to sex. They may have failed to consider the possibility that what many men want most—their own penis thrusting inside a vagina—is not necessarily what women want most.

4
Male Identification

Dora insisted that she was not attracted to Herr K. and even said that Herr K.'s efforts to seduce her had filled her with disgust. But Freud believed he knew better: "This was truly just the situation to call up a distinct feeling of sexual excitement in a girl of [thirteen]." He presumed that an adolescent girl who rejects the sexual overtures of a married man more than twice her age (a man not unlike Freud himself) has to be neurotic. To all appearances, Freud was viewing Dora the way a heterosexual man sees a woman, as an erotic object, but also as a lesser object, a person less deserving, less worthy, and entitled. This heterosexual male perspective continued to dominate the sex therapy discipline that Freudian psychology spawned, prevailing even when female therapists treated their patients.

That a female therapist can have the kind of pro-male, anti-female biases that characterized Freud's practice is at once surprising and a phenomenon of growing importance, as the field of psychotherapy and the subfield of sex therapy have become increasingly dominated by female practitioners.[1] Kathleen Barry described the configuration of these kinds of biases as a world view in which "women place men above women, including themselves, in credibility, status, and importance in most situations, regardless of the comparative quality the women may bring to the situation."[2] Barry labeled this world view "male identification." In it, women, as well as men, operate as if the world and everything in it exist primarily for men, while women have been designed by nature for the singular purpose of serving men.

Helen Singer Kaplan

Although not as well known to the public as Masters and Johnson, Helen Singer Kaplan was, in some ways, as influential, through her advocacy of Masters and Johnson's treatment formulations in over one hundred books and papers, her tutelage of sex therapists at the Cornell University Medical School, the first medical school in the United States with its own sex therapy clinic,[3] and her efforts to promote inhibited sexual desire as a psychiatric issue, the sexual disorder that soon became the most common problem women presented to therapists.[4] What I wish to explore in this chapter is how Kaplan, like Freud and Masters and Johnson, may have pressured women to accept masculine versions of sexual normality—how she may have projected pro-male, anti-female biases onto her female patients—and in so doing, encouraged them to admit that, deep down, despite their repeated denials, what they really wanted and needed is a penis, their husband's penis, thrusting inside their vagina.

While Kaplan acknowledged that "society fosters female dependency and male exploitation: guilt in girls about achievement and guilt in boys about failure to achieve,"[5] she did not believe that women were disadvantaged. Accordingly, Kaplan's professional record shows little attention to signs of male privilege and dominance. She explained gender inequality as a wash: "These gender assignments are exceedingly harmful to *both* genders, not only in the area of sexual functioning, but in all areas of life as well. . . . The male is no better off."[6] Despite this assertion, Kaplan maintained that the sexual deck is stacked against men because of their *inborn* disadvantages, noting that men are slower sexual learners than women and less able to control their sexual impulses. Kaplan thus reasoned that, because nature endowed men with a sex drive that is much more powerful and "compelling" than women's, it is "less subject to inhibition by learning than the female's sex drive."[7] Perhaps this explains her partiality to male reasoning, an inclination philosopher Kate Manne called "himpathy."[8] Kaplan might have aspired to work out equitable compromises between men and women in conflict over sexual issues, but as the next case study reveals, her analysis and treatment were often grounded in her male patients' point of view.

The Myth of Equivalency

To provide some background information on this case which originally appeared in Kaplan's *Sexual Aversion, Sexual Phobias, and Panic Disorders* (1987), the husband, Norman, was sixty-five, a retired attorney, and his wife, Norma, age fifty, was a successful artist. At the time they began treatment, Norman and Norma had not had sex in several months, with Norman claiming that his wife "had grown distant and disinterested." However, when Kaplan, in an effort to get the couple's love life back on track, asked them to perform daily sexual exercises at home, they hit a snag. Norman and Norma could not do their homework because, as he explained, his wife refused to make love in the early mornings, the time of day he preferred having sex. Norma tried to clarify why sex in the early mornings did not work well for her. She said she would be happy to make love with Norman at any other time, but she reserved her early mornings for painting, the time of day when her creativity peaked. That explanation not only failed to satisfy Norman; it infuriated him. This is how Kaplan described his reaction:

The husband could not contain his smoldering rage. His wife's involvement with her work tapped into old feelings of pain and anger about having been slighted and "ignored" by his career-oriented mother. He developed insomnia and behaved irritably and badly towards Norma all week.[9]

A therapist could respond to Norman's rage in any number of ways. For instance, a therapist might suggest, ever so gently, that Norman needed to get over it. A therapist might suggest that he was overreacting and that if he was serious about wanting Norma to become less "distant and disinterested," he might take more of an interest in her creativity and career. A therapist might also ask him to imagine how he would respond if his wife asked him, before he retired from his law firm, not to go into work during the time of day when his most important meetings were scheduled, as a favor to her, because that happened to be the time she most needed his companionship. A therapist might ask him to consider that Norma's career means as much to her as his once meant to him.

But there is no record of Kaplan's having entertained such possibilities. What she did suggest, according to the case study, is a compromise. While Kaplan acknowledged that "many artists do their best work before the pressures of the day interrupt their thoughts and that [Norma's] habit of painting in the morning was not a rejection of [Norman]," she also pointed out that Norman's desire for sex in the morning "was not just a means of bullying her." Kaplan explained that "men at his age function best in the early morning on a physical basis and that it was quite natural that he would want sex at that time."[10] In other words, she proposed that both parties give in a little. Norman could sacrifice his morning sex four times a week so Norma could paint, and Norma could sacrifice her morning painting three times a week, so Norman could have sex.

It seemed a reasonable solution, except that the "compromise" is based on a false equivalence, an issue Arlie Hochschild examined in her study of working parents, *The Second Shift*. One of Hochschild's cases involved Nancy Holt, a wife who arrived home from her full-time job as a social worker only to perform a second full-time shift at home, where she was responsible for almost all the housework and childcare. Naturally, she felt overwhelmed and exploited. However, when she asked her husband to share the burden with her, he balked, and the conflict started to affect their sex life. Nancy told her husband, "Look Evan, I would not be this exhausted and asexual every night if I didn't have so much to face every morning."[11] She considered separating, but not for very long because she became frightened, and her fear prompted her to see the world as she imagined a man might see it. "Why wreck a marriage over a dirty frying pan?" she asked herself. "Evan was 'so good' in other ways . . . women always adjust more, don't they?" Then, to make the unfairness of the marriage arrangement less painful, dropping any and all misgivings about "male identification," she developed what amounts to a delusional system centered on a myth of equivalence. She decided that her responsibility for the "upstairs" chores (the meals, childcare, shopping, cleaning, etc.) was the moral equivalent of Evan's "downstairs" chores (the garage, the basement workshop, dog care). Through the fiction that they each shared responsibility for half the house, Nancy, a feminist, managed to suppress her resentment and imagine that her arrangement with Evan was egalitarian.[12]

Equating Norman's desire for sex in the morning with Norma's desire to pursue her career as a painter represents a similar mythology. Both were created to allow a woman to pretend that her marriage is egalitarian. The difference, what makes Kaplan's "compromise" between Norma and Norman appear even more unfair and extreme, is that, while women are routinely asked to perform a disproportionate share of housework in addition to their career responsibilities, as was true of Nancy Holt, it's nearly impossible to imagine a husband asking, no less demanding, that his wife take time off from work so she can provide sexual services for him. This is where Kaplan's "himpathy" appears most transparent: not only was Kaplan unmoved by this kind of social, structural inequality, she badgered Norma to accept it. Consider, for example, that Kaplan's efforts to make Norma appreciate the depth of "Norman's pain and his fury at feeling that he was playing second fiddle to his wife's work," included introducing the notion that Norman had an "inherent sensitivity to rejections," all because he believed that his mother preferred her career to him.[13] Kaplan took the position that Norma, whom Norman brought to therapy because he believed she had lost sexual interest in him, needed to sacrifice an important part of her career to help her husband manage his sexual/emotional insecurities. Norman needed Norma to make that sacrifice, Kaplan explained, because her commitment to her career "tapped into his old pain and anger."

What Kaplan does not appear to have considered is how important Norma's creativity was to her. Neither did she consider that, by tapping into Norma's feelings of fear, obligation, and responsibility in this way—by activating her "old unresolved guilt about putting her own needs before those of others"[14]—she may have compromised Norma's capacity for sexual consent. Kaplan probably did not imagine that she could have been holding an emotional bludgeon over Norma's head by suggesting, in effect, "Either you provide Norman with sex at the times that work best for him, or you will be held responsible for the poor man's psychological collapse."

Men's Sexual Sensitivity

Sex therapy for heterosexual couples, in general, posits a man's need for sex as inherently normal and functional, while positing a woman's lack of interest in sex at the times he wants, and in the ways he wants, as inherently abnormal and dysfunctional. That's why case studies describing a husband who feels sexually neglected tend to focus on getting his wife to "improve" her sexual performance. Such a focus explains the frequent appearance in the professional literature of case studies in which "success" is achieved when the wife's sexual behavior becomes aligned with her husband's sexual needs. It's a matter of his right and her obligation. Here's how Joe, aged thirty-one, married eleven years, explained this kind of asymmetric arrangement to researchers studying the performance of sex in long-term heterosexual relationships. Note, in particular, Joe's description of his wife's cooperative attitude and his claim that she recognizes that his feelings of sexual deprivation are not just a problem for him, but a problem for her. It's something she needs to fix:

> I'm sort of hypersensitive about it. I easily feel rejected. And so I let her know.... I've let her know over the years.... It's usually me that brings it up whenever our sex life is screwed up in some way or declining or whatever. And the reaction is rarely hostile. It's usually that, by the time I'm bringing it up, she is starting to become aware of it and realizes that, you know, we need to fix it.[15]

Much of this gender imbalance is due to the same kind of social conventions that govern a waiter's obligations to a diner. Most of us have been schooled to understand that when we are dining out, we have reason to complain when our waiter keeps us waiting for an inordinate period and then serves our food in an unfriendly, disagreeable manner. We understand this is bad service. Similarly, according to prevailing sexual conventions, we often judge a wife who does not provide her husband with timely, attentive sexual service as negligent. We judge her to be in violation of her tacit, although fundamental, sex role obligations. As Dworkin explained, "she is his; not flesh of his flesh at all in terms of rights or dignity of being but belonging to him in sex, his authority over her expressed in his sexual rights over her, which, in the end, are absolute."[16] Although, perhaps, not *rigidly* absolute, since people usually make exceptions for temporary indispositions such as illness or injury. However, if she does not eventually come around, for whatever reason, her husband is often seen as the injured party, the one deserving sympathy, and she is judged as the wrongdoer, the one needing some form of correction or sanction. Breanne Fahs and Eric Swank (2016), in their research on "women's emotion work in their sexual relationships" call this asymmetric obligation, women's "other third shift:" the time required for women to take care of men's sexual needs in much the same manner they are required to take care of men's housework needs through "the second shift."[17]

In keeping with the expectations of the "other third shift," if a husband complains to a sex therapist that his wife has been neglecting him in bed, it's

78   BIRTH OF SEX THERAPY

likely that he'll find support,[18] which is more or less what happened in a case study Kaplan presented in *The New Sex Therapy* (1974) involving a man suffering from "premature ejaculation." The wife complained of feeling dehumanized by the obligation to service what she perceived as her husband's mechanical, impersonal sexual needs, but from what is reported in the case study, Kaplan pays little attention to these objections. Instead, Kaplan seemed to encourage her to continue servicing him the way he preferred.

WIFE: It's so mechanical—just stimulating his penis. I get tired . . . it's so artificial . . . it's not really romantic. The whole thing is very disappointing.

KAPLAN: It really sounds as if it were tedious for you.

WIFE: It certainly is. My hand gets tired, and he just lies there and does nothing. I'm very discouraged.

KAPLAN: I'm sorry to hear that. I thought that he was attaining pretty good control last week, didn't you?

HUSBAND: Oh, yes, doctor, I can really feel the difference. I'm very encouraged, I never held out so long before.

KAPLAN: Well that's a shame then. Just when treatment seems to be working out, you [*the wife*] get tired of it.

WIFE: Well, it's so artificial and mechanical. There's no love involved.

KAPLAN: I can really see your point; it's not much fun for you. Do you want to stop treatment?

WIFE: Well, I don't know. . . . After all, I'm not a mechanical robot. . . . I want pleasure too. I mean how long is this going to go on . . . will I have to jerk him off forever? [*to the husband*] What do *you* want to do?

HUSBAND: Well, I . . . I don't want to stop . . . well I don't know . . . I enjoy it . . . but I don't know. Whatever you want dear.

WIFE [*to Kaplan*]: Isn't there something else we could do? How long does this go on?

KAPLAN: If you recall, at our first session I told you it usually takes about three weeks of practice before the man's control is good enough for satisfactory intercourse. To answer your first question, no . . . I'm afraid I don't know any other method that works. I know that the procedure may get a bit tedious for the woman and I don't blame you for wanting to stop. In fact, I think you should stop, because he is a very sensitive man and now he probably senses your reluctance, so it may not work in any case.[19]

Kaplan cited the husband's sensitivity as a reason for the wife to service him willingly and congenially in much the same way she cited Norman's sensitivities when trying to convince Norma to acquiesce to his sexual demands. In her accounts of the two cases, Kaplan expressed no comparable concern for the wife's sensitivities. In an effort to reassure the wife who feared she would have to jerk her husband off forever, Kaplan said that if she could hang in and resist the impulse to quit, she and her husband would soon be getting to satisfying intercourse. *I told you it usually takes about three weeks of practice before the man's control is good enough for satisfactory intercourse.* Kaplan does not acknowledge that intercourse is not what the wife was asking for; she was asking for a type of sex that required her husband to treat her as a person. What the wife objected to, and what Kaplan did not overtly support or acknowledge, is the artificiality and impersonality—the fundamental one-sidedness—of what she had to do for her husband's pleasure ("There's no love involved").

A Wife in Bondage

I included the case articulating the wife's perhaps unpleasant obligation to service her husband's sexual needs for the same reason I included the Norma–Norman case. Both reveal Kaplan's privileging a man's sexual needs over those of his wife. One might argue that in the Norma–Norman case, the wife's needs were acknowledged, at least in part. In the compromise Kaplan worked out, Norma may have been pressured to acquiesce to Norman's sexual demands, but she still got to paint four mornings a week. In the next case study, also from Kaplan's, *The New Sex Therapy*, even partial acknowledgement of the woman's needs is absent.

This case involves a twenty-eight-year-old stay at home mother married to a thirty-eight-year-old physician. The presenting problem, according to Kaplan, "was the wife's growing reluctance to have intercourse with her husband. He had always had a strong sex drive and wanted to have intercourse frequently, usually every day."[20] In this case, the most graphic illustration of the sex therapist's failure to recognize male privilege and dominance occurred in Kaplan's response to this couple's failed attempt to carry off their sensate focus exercise. As the partners were engaging in this exercise, the wife reported that she "suddenly 'turned off' and asked her husband to stop. He became furious, shouted at her, and accused her of being spoiled, demanding, and unreasonable,"[21] a response mode (a husband's direct expression of anger during or immediately following sex) that researchers have found especially distressing to women who report sexual dysfunctions.[22] Instead of judiciously informing the husband that he was wrong to lose his temper and call his wife names—instead of warning him against behaving like a tyrant—Kaplan suggested that it was a bad idea for the wife to refuse to follow her husband's sexual lead. To emphasize the importance of this message, Kaplan reports that she "directly confronted [the wife] with the fact that she seemed to actively avoid being 'turned on' sexually,"[23] framing sexual excitement as an act of will. Instead of "confronting" a husband about losing his temper with his wife during sex, she scolded the wife for "the fact" that she was willfully resisting sex with her husband. Because she did not regard the wife as the victim of a sexually bullying husband, she blamed the wife's resistance for the sexual conflict, conveying the message that it is normal or acceptable for a husband to yell at and abuse his wife when she does not respond to his sexual initiatives in the ways he wants.

As the couple's therapy progressed, the wife revealed that she continued to have trouble responding to her husband sexually because she did not feel fully committed to their marriage. As she described her feelings to Kaplan, she represented her marriage as a kind of "bondage." She told Kaplan that in return for financial support, she felt "she had to 'service' her husband, to devote herself to his well-being, and to give up any active creative career goals of her own."[24] Kaplan acknowledges that the wife's perceptions are real and not delusional, reporting that the husband had "a similar image of their roles and relationship."[25] The wife may, of course, have entered into this asymmetric power arrangement with her head up; she may have understood from the beginning of her marriage that she would be obligated to devote herself to her husband's needs, in exchange for his financial support, as a servant or prostitute might. But that does not mean that it was not extremely harmful. As the case study reveals, Kaplan did not respond to the wife's "bondage" revelation as if it represented a serious problem, requiring direct intervention or even inquiry. Kaplan raised no questions about the feelings of a woman in a marriage that obligated her to engage in unpleasurable, undesired sex at her husband's command. She did not question how this position might affect the wife's autonomy, pride, and sense of self. Instead, the case study seems to interpret the wife's sad resignation as a rebellious willfulness and shifts attention from the topic of "bondage" by vaguely noting that "alternative viewpoints and solutions were explored in treatment" and that, although as therapy progressed, the wife "was still ambivalent about her marriage, she was able to make the decision to improve her sex life, which she no longer equated with a lifelong irrevocable commitment to the bondage of matrimony."[26]

Although the husband became enraged when he felt his sexual needs were not being properly serviced, the case study does not present him as having a sexual or psychological problem, nor does it ever refer to him as a "patient." Perhaps because he had a strong sexual appetite, perhaps because he wanted sex daily, and perhaps because he fits the cultural ideal of the sexually dominant male,[27] he figures in this case as sexually normal. By contrast, because his wife had little interest in sex, often pleading headaches and fatigue in response to her husband's sexual advances, she is presented as the official "patient."

Today, we might see the wife as the victim of gender domination and the logic of Kaplan's treatment method as blaming the victim. Kaplan's case study frames the wife's recovery as doing the husband's bidding. However, in addition to physical compliance, Kaplan wanted her patient to express signs of sexual arousal as she went along with his demands. Thus, in the end, Kaplan reported this case as a treatment success because "the couple worked out a mutually arousing and satisfactory tempo and style of lovemaking which resulted in the patient's increased responsiveness and lowered orgastic threshold."[28] To translate: although the wife continued in a fundamentally unequal relationship and continued to imagine herself in bondage, she was reporting orgasms at least once in a while. In Kaplan's opinion, she was finally getting something out of sex. "Moreover," Kaplan went on, "she was able to resolve the conflict between her need to be independent and her desire for a close 'dependent' relationship, at least to some degree."[29] To translate: she wasn't complaining about her bondage as much.

Sexual Anorexia

Like Freud and Masters and Johnson, Kaplan argued that sexual inhibition occurs when anxiety or fear becomes associated with sexual activity. But instead of likening the sex drive to a flowing stream that seeks to return to its natural stream bed, she likened it to a feeling of hunger—a feeling of nutritional deprivation. By implication, for Kaplan, the sexually inhibited or sexually inactive woman is not merely frustrated; she is starving. This is more than a rhetorical distinction. If forgoing nutriment by deliberately and continually conjuring up noxious associations to food indicates a most serious psychiatric dysfunction, anorexia nervosa, then, for Kaplan, forgoing sexual activity by deliberately and continually conjuring up noxious associations to sex indicates an analogous psychiatric dysfunction, "sexual anorexia":

> My observations of patients with "sexual anorexia" or HSD [hypoactive sexual desire] indicate that the psychogenic form of this syndrome is caused by their active, albeit unconscious selectively negative cognitive and perceptual processes by means of which they literally "turn themselves off." In other words, while normal persons "accentuate the positives, and decentuate the negatives" (to borrow from Johnny Mercer's famous lyrics), in order to maximize their sexual arousal and pleasure, patients with HSD inappropriately suppress their sexual feelings by dwelling on their partners' negative qualities, while they "decentuate the positives," that is, blind themselves to their attractive features.[30]

Kaplan acknowledged that people's reasons for "turning themselves off" sexually can sometimes be realistic and adaptive, as when they are confronted by dangerous or threatening sexual situations. Under more normal circumstances, however, Kaplan considered sexual inhibition to be pathological. She explained that this pathology occurs "when the patient does not feel desire for an attractive and appropriate partner; when desire is dampened by unprovoked anger, by mistrust for a spouse who is in reality giving and loving."[31] The challenge for Kaplan, as well as for other sex therapists, is how to determine what constitutes an "attractive" and "appropriate" partner, who is "giving and loving." How can therapists determine whether a patient's sexual disinterest is normal or pathological, except through recourse to their own sexual predilections? How does a therapist judge a woman patient who appears to have no sexual interest in a husband whom the therapist finds "attractive" and "appropriate"?

This is the challenge Kaplan faced in another case reported in *The New Sex Therapy* involving the M.'s, a married couple in their mid-thirties with a baby. Mrs. M. did not find her husband attractive and had almost no interest in having sex with him, but Kaplan disagreed, or at least had a very different reaction to Mr. M. She described him as "a strikingly handsome, charming, well-spoken man, who moved with grace."[32] By contrast, she found Mrs. M. decidedly unattractive: "Although the wife had good features, her unbecoming hair-style, lack of makeup, and unattractive clothes made her appear homely. Moreover, her posture was bad, and her movements were tense and constricted."[33] Kaplan's account of this case suggests that the wife should be delighted to have sex with such an attractive man and therefore dismisses as bogus every reason Mrs. M. gave for her sexual disinterest in him.[34]

To illustrate, at the initial interview, Mrs. M. made two startling admissions. First, she "ascribed her inability to respond to her husband sexually to the fact that she did not love him." Second, "she claimed she was in love with another man."[35] Many therapists would say that admissions of this kind should be taken very seriously and should be explored with a host of follow-up questions such as, "Did you ever love your husband?" and if the answer is "yes," they might try to establish what changed. They might also ask, why, if Mrs. M. doesn't love her husband, she is still with him, and perhaps most important, why, if she loves someone else, she is now in sex therapy with her husband, attempting to improve their sexual relationship. Kaplan does not report those questions in the case study. Instead, she describes how she began prescribing a series of sensate focus exercises for the couple that included "caressing each other's bodies" and "lightly [stimulating] each other's genitals."[36]

At the third session, the couple reported that the results of these exercises had been extremely positive: "For the first time since her adolescence, Mrs. M. experienced some erotic feelings and felt elated about this."[37] However, when they were seen the following week—the fourth session—they were both very discouraged. In each of the three times that Mr. M. attempted to have sex with his wife,

Mrs. M. had been unresponsive. Mrs. M. explained why she had been unresponsive by referring to the temperature of the bedroom. The coldness "sort of ruined the whole thing," she said. A second excuse concerned their child: "The baby was up, and mother was downstairs, and it was too much trouble." The third excuse, as the husband reported, was a bit more complicated: "I started to touch her and I got really excited and she seemed really turned on. Then she made me stop all of a sudden. She turned on the lights and checked the bed. She thought her period started—and that sort of interrupted things. I got really mad." This is the conversation that followed:

MRS. M.: Well I was so wet. I just thought I must have messed up the bed. I did give you an orgasm, so what are you mad about?
MR. M.: Well I didn't stay mad.
KAPLAN: I'd like to hear more about what happened.
MRS. M.: I know . . . Well, I really started to feel good . . . and Ted was very excited . . . and I felt all wet down there. Then, all of a sudden I thought, "Oh my God I'm bleeding all over the bed. My mother will really get mad at me" [they were staying at her mother's house at the time] . . . I just had to check it out, and I was really surprised . . . it was okay. And Ted yelled at me, and then everything was, like over. Later we talked, and then I gave him an orgasm.
KAPLAN: Did you try again the next day?
MRS. M.: No . . . no we didn't. We didn't do anything for the rest of the week.
KAPLAN [*to Mrs. M.*]: It seems to me that you find some way to turn yourself off when you feel sexually aroused.
MRS. M.: No I don't. I really thought I had messed up the bed . . . and before, it was really cold. I couldn't help it.
MR. M.: Oh honey! Come on . . . of course you do . . . the doctor's right.
MRS. M.: No . . . well I just . . . it just happens . . . maybe you are right. But why? Why would I do that?
KAPLAN: I don't know—maybe you get anxious when you feel aroused. It's an important question. We should work on it.[38]

To all appearances, Mr. M. and Mrs. M. offered completely different accounts of what had ruined their most recent sexual efforts. While Mrs. M. argued that circumstances beyond her control interfered with her capacity to respond sexually (the coldness of the room, the baby fussing, the possibility that her mother's sheets would become messed, and her husband yelling at her), her husband countered that none of them interfered with his capacity to respond sexually. "It wasn't that cold," he said. "I wasn't cold." Nor was he distracted by the baby fussing or by the possibility that they would be blamed for staining the sheets. He also said his yelling shouldn't be treated as a big issue. "I didn't stay mad," he said.

None of these circumstances had distracted him from sex. Why then should his wife be distracted? What was her problem?

Arbitrating this dispute in a gender-neutral way, without pro-male bias, might involve acknowledging that people often have different sensitivities to cold and that someone might not want to take her clothes off when she's shivering. Another acknowledgement might be that mothers and fathers often have different reactions to the sound of a baby crying. Furthermore, as a cultural norm, a woman might be more distracted from sex by the fear she might be staining another woman's linen. As for Mr. M.'s yelling, a gender-neutral perspective might have acknowledged that, although Mr. M. didn't take his yelling very seriously, his wife did. After all, they were not just attempting to stimulate each other's genital organs, they were attempting to make love. A lot of women, and a lot of men, too, withdraw from lovemaking when their partners yell at them.

Kaplan's report, however, does not position the therapist in the role of gender-neutral arbiter. Instead, she appeared to handle Mrs. M.'s explanations for her lack of sexual follow-through as she handled Mrs. M.'s confession that she did not love her husband and as she responded to the wife's complaint in the previous case that her marriage represented a kind of "bondage." In both instances, Kaplan simply moved on. Mrs. M.'s sexual problems, as Kaplan saw them, were all in her head. In Kaplan's words, "It seems to me that you find some way to turn yourself off when you feel sexually excited." Similarly, Kaplan reports that she "directly confronted" the wife who complained of being held in bondage: "with the fact that she seemed to actively avoid being 'turned on' sexually."

Shortly after this juncture, when Kaplan concluded that Mrs. M.'s sexual reticence was not responding to the mix of exercises that she prescribed for the couple, she decided to take a more psychoanalytic, Freudian approach to Mrs. M.'s treatment. Accordingly, she began seeing Mrs. M. alone, in individual therapy, which had as its focus Mrs. M.'s childhood and her relationship with her mother, as well as her other allegedly "deep" intrapsychic issues. Mrs. M., a woman who claimed to be in love with another man—a woman who claimed she did not love, or wish to have sex with, her "strikingly handsome" husband—had become, according to Kaplan's case study, the sex therapy equivalent of a madwoman. Kaplan constituted Mrs. M.'s resistance to change as a problem of exceptional psychopathology, requiring intense one-on-one intervention, the guiding purpose of which was to uncover the patient's underlying reasons for resisting intercourse with her "attractive" and "appropriate" husband on his terms, in the ways he wanted and at the times most convenient to him.

In failing to recognize the ways men's sexual needs are culturally privileged, Kaplan perhaps unwittingly supported that cultural bias. One of the ways she may have done this was to set an uncommonly low bar for what constitutes an "attractive" and "appropriate" male sex partner and, by implication, an uncommonly low bar for a woman's sexual pathology, as evidenced by her choice of the starvation metaphor for sexual inhibition. If, for a woman suffering from anorexia nervosa, calories from a Twinkie are preferable to total fasting, then for a woman suffering from "sexual anorexia," sex with almost any man, in almost any circumstance, is a healthier choice than complete abstinence. This should become clearer in the next case example taken from Kaplan's *The Sexual Desire Disorders* (1995), which illustrates how Kaplan diagnosed and treated a young woman's reluctance to have intercourse even under the most disadvantageous, disempowering conditions.

A Prisoner of Sex

Esther, aged eighteen, and Shlomo, aged nineteen, members of an Orthodox Jewish sect, had been married three months when Esther began seeing Kaplan. Esther's marriage to Shlomo had been arranged by their families, and Esther had only met Shlomo once, briefly, before signing the marriage contract. On their wedding night, after Esther and Shlomo had intercourse, she broke into uncontrollable sobs. It was not because the intercourse had been painful. She said that Shlomo had been neither brutal nor inconsiderate, and she confessed that she could not fully account for the depth of her despair. Nonetheless, since her wedding night she had developed feelings of loathing and aversion to Shlomo that were so intense, she could not bear being in the same house with him. She found the sight of him intolerable.[39]

To test the intensity of Esther's aversion, Kaplan asked her to evaluate Shlomo from a distance—to look at him from the screened women's balcony of the synagogue while Shlomo was at prayer on the ground floor—and then report back on how this made her feel. Esther did as she was told, and reported that "the mere sight of Shlomo precipitated a severe panic attack and [she] had to be taken from the synagogue."[40]

For their next therapy session, Kaplan asked Esther to bring a photo of her husband. According to Kaplan, "the snapshot depicted a tall, thin, fine-looking young man with a full dark beard in typical Hasidic garb." Kaplan remarked to Esther, "He looks kind of handsome to me. What is it you don't like about Shlomo?" In response, Esther rose to her feet, spat on the picture, tore it to pieces, threw the pieces to the floor, and then stomped on them. Consistent with Katherine Hayles's argument that the only normal and acceptable voice for a woman in a male world is a voice that does not directly express hostility,[41] Kaplan interpreted Esther's angry outburst as a sign of the most severe psychopathy: "Esther's sexual aversion to her husband was clearly pathological," and therefore warranted a proportionally severe diagnosis, "sexual aversion disorder with concomitant panic disorder."

The most remarkable feature of this brief vignette is that it took several sessions before Kaplan got around to asking Esther, "What is it you don't like about Shlomo?" The failure to ask a woman her reasons for rejecting her partner, when that rejection is what prompts therapy, is hard to explain except on the grounds that the therapist had already made up her mind about Shlomo and Esther. Kaplan may have assumed, from the outset, that the wife had no valid reasons for rejecting her husband. Although Kaplan never met with Shlomo, she described him as not only "fine looking" and "handsome," but also as "a gifted 19-year-old Talmudic scholar . . . the eldest son of distinguished rabbi."[42] On the other hand, she had nothing positive to say about Esther. Once again, Kaplan implied that the husband was a good catch—attractive and appropriate—and that the wife's rejection of him appeared pathological.

Kaplan only asked Esther, "What is it you don't like about him?" after she had openly declared that Shlomo "looks kind of handsome to me," a comment that seemed to convey bafflement as to why Esther was fussing so much about this man. Kaplan's comment also fails to consider Esther's youth, the fact that she was only eighteen, as a matter of great concern. Nor does the case foreground the forced nature of Esther's marriage, which obliged her to have intercourse with Shlomo, a complete stranger up to the point of their wedding, to bear and raise his children—to share her entire life with him. Kaplan defended her belief that Esther needed psychiatric treatment by affirming her cultural norms as appropriate and right for Esther: "If [Esther] were to have a future in a community that accepted nothing less than marriage and motherhood for their women, she would have to undergo treatment to overcome her aversion to sex."[43] From these comments, Kaplan appeared to recognize that Esther's community was oppressive, but that did not alarm Kaplan, according to the text, as much as Esther's rebellion. The pathology Kaplan finally treats in this case is Esther's autonomy, her refusal to accept her subordinate position in her community—her refusal to accept the life that others had arranged for her.

Kaplan's professional male identification is further revealed in a comparable case, also from her book, *The Sexual Desire Disorders*, in which the sexually reticent patient was a man. That case also involves an arranged marriage in which a spouse could not go through with intercourse, despite the other partner's willingness and the family's insistence. In the latter case, Dr. Raj, the spouse who lacked sexual desire, was "a handsome, tall, 32-year-old physician from Bombay." He could not become aroused enough to maintain an erection with his new wife, and, as a consequence, every attempt at intercourse failed. However, unlike Esther and Shlomo's failed marriage, the explanation turned out to be fairly simple, at least to Kaplan: "The trouble which Dr. Raj revealed to me in private was that he was deeply in love with another woman, a beautiful, tall, blonde, athletic physician.... The doctor didn't know it, but he was acting out his desire to remain faithful to the woman he loved."[44]

The inconsistency is hard to miss. Why did Kaplan find a young woman's negative response to her arranged marriage symptomatic of a profound psychiatric disorder, but a man's negative reaction to his arranged marriage entirely reasonable? Why did Kaplan readily accept this man's love for another woman as an explanation for his situational lack of desire but, to all appearances, found it impossible to accept an identical explanation from a woman, Mrs. M., for her lack of desire for her husband?

One possibility is that in cases such as these, when women's accounts of their sexual experiences are discredited, dismissed, and ignored, it is not simply that the facts of women's sex lives are rendered "not known," it is that women, as members of a disadvantaged group, are rendered "not knowers."[45] Women are constructed as less knowledgeable than men, less truthful, less conscious, and overall, as less credible. A second possibility has to do with therapists' perceived obligation to uphold society's dominant ideologies.[46] In that role, they represent and mirror societal conceptions of normality—in particular, male identification. A husband, therefore, as a man, is seen as deserving greater license, in general, to do as he pleases sexually, which includes greater license to be excused from the obligation to engage in unwanted, unpleasurable intercourse with his spouse. As we shall see in the chapters that follow, a husband's lack of desire for his wife is more likely to be seen as rational and, hence, as more pardonable than his wife's lack of desire for him. A wife may have an obligation to consent to sex whether she wants it or not, but no reciprocal obligation exists for a husband who is entitled to have as much or as little sex as he wants.

5
Docile Bodies

Having explained to the patient the nature of her flinching, she must be taught how to maintain the best posture for coitus and how to achieve relaxation of the sphincter muscles. She must be helped to see for herself that hyperaesthesia is a fiction and that pain is of her own making. She must be trained to tolerate the entry of the examining finger and later self-inserted vaginal dilators. No frightened woman is going to like these procedures, but, curiously, she will respond better to firmness than too much sympathy.
—Joan Malleson, "Sex Problems in Marriage" (1954)

The following sex therapy exercise involves a therapist asking a male patient to imagine what it would feel like to put his penis next to his wife's vagina—"right up to the opening."[1]

THERAPIST: It feels okay there?
HUSBAND: Yes, it is still erect.
THERAPIST: All right, then let us slowly move it in. Let us move it in barely an eighth of an inch, so that it is barely in. How does that feel?
HUSBAND: That feels good.
THERAPIST: Is that all right? How about a little more, maybe half an inch? Is that all right?
HUSBAND: That still feels good.
THERAPIST: Still erect? How about moving it an inch? That feels good still?
HUSBAND: It is erect and feels good but there is a sense of a threat coming back.
THERAPIST: Then we will come back out again. Bring it out. Okay, let us see if we can move it in a little bit again. Get it in about an eighth of an inch? Okay there?
HUSBAND: Yes, it is fine there.
THERAPIST: Okay, how about half an inch?
HUSBAND: It is still fine.
THERAPIST: Bring it in an inch now. Can you get it in an inch?
HUSBAND: It's still okay.
THERAPIST: All right, an inch and a half?

HUSBAND: It is still okay.
THERAPIST: Two inches?
HUSBAND: Now there is a little...
THERAPIST: Okay, let us take it out slowly. Now do you still have an erection?
HUSBAND: Yes.
THERAPIST: Okay, let us try again. Half an inch? An inch?
HUSBAND: It still feels nice.
THERAPIST: An inch and a half?
HUSBAND: It still feels good.
THERAPIST: A couple of inches now?
HUSBAND: It feels a lot better.
THERAPIST: Two and a half inches?
HUSBAND: It still feels good.
THERAPIST: Three inches?
HUSBAND: It still feels good.
THERAPIST: Three and a half inches?
HUSBAND: It still feels good.
THERAPIST: Four inches?
HUSBAND: It feels a lot better now.
THERAPIST: Four and a half inches now?
HUSBAND: It feels very good.
THERAPIST: Five inches?
HUSBAND: It still feels good.
THERAPIST: Can you put it in all the way now? Can you see how it feels?
HUSBAND: It feels really neat.

At this point in the exercise, the therapist began asking the husband to imagine himself moving his penis slowly in and out of his wife's vagina. After the husband complied, the therapist asked him how he felt about it, and as before, the husband said it feels "good" and "really good." As these positive responses continued, the therapist eventually gave the husband permission to become aggressive: "Okay, now you can thrust, continue to thrust back and forth." This was followed by the therapist asking, "Feel the power of the thrust? How do you feel?" to which the husband replied, "It feels really nice."

THERAPIST: It feels very, very powerful?
HUSBAND: Yes, powerful.
THERAPIST: Very, very powerful?
HUSBAND: It feels affection...
 Therapist? Very, very potent?
HUSBAND: Yes.

THERAPIST: Very, very masculine?
HUSBAND: Yes.
THERAPIST: Very, very fulfilling?
HUSBAND: It does feel that, yes.[2]

This sex therapy exercise can be compared to the ether-induced coma of the English wife whose sexual story began this book; they are comparable even though more than a century separates them. A continent also separates them, since the sex therapy exercise took place in Long Beach, California, at the Center for Marital and Sexual Studies. Another difference is that, in the case of the English woman, there was actual copulation, while in the therapy exercise, there was nothing more than a fantasy. In the former, a therapeutic intervention was directed to the woman, requiring the inhalation of ether. In the latter, a therapeutic intervention was directed only to the man.

Still, among so many differences, there is a striking similarity: the absence of an active, conscious, responsive woman. In both the ether-induced and the imaginary copulation, the sexual experience was entirely one-sided. The English woman was blacked out; the ether made her insensible. In the case of the American man's copulation fantasy, his wife may as well have been blacked out, since his thoughts were focused exclusively on his penis, how it felt, and how he felt about it, inside his wife's vagina. At one point, the husband referred to feelings of affection ("It feels affection . . ."), but the therapist immediately cut him off. Other than that, he had absolutely nothing to say about the person with whom he was supposedly sharing this experience, an absence that can be attributed as much to the therapist as to the husband, for at no point did the therapist encourage him to speculate on how his wife might be responding. In short, in both the ethereal copulation and the imaginary copulation, the woman appeared as nothing more than an object on whom the husband could perform at will. In neither situation was attention paid to the possible meanings vaginal penetration had for the woman. No attention was paid to the question of whether she might feel satisfied or dissatisfied, comfortable or uncomfortable, or, indeed, whether she had any needs of her own which might, in some way, impact this experience, and influence their interaction. The emphasis was on one person's experience—the man's.[3]

Here are some additional differences: the linkage between power and intercourse implied in the ether-induced copulation became explicit in the therapy exercise. In asking the husband whether he felt "powerful," "potent," and "masculine," the therapist was encouraging the husband to imagine himself exercising power over another person, his wife, the object of his power, the receptacle of his thrusting. Furthermore, the therapist encouraged the husband to imagine feelings of pleasure in this exercise of power. In performing the exercise under the guidance of the therapist, the husband learned that it is appropriate to dominate his wife through intercourse and to take pleasure in that domination. Sexual domination is supposed to feel good. It's supposed to feel "very, very fulfilling."[4]

The therapists who designed the copulation exercise, William Hartman and Marilyn Fithian, were known as "Masters and Johnson West,"[5] because they shared a number of Masters and Johnson's beliefs: first, that sexual experience is best understood in terms of physical sensation, sensory pleasure, and relief from sexual tension; second, that only the sexual dysfunction should be targeted for change in sex therapy; third, that sexual healing should not take very long; fourth, that healing can be facilitated by asking patients to participate in a series of highly structured sexual exercises; and fifth, the Freudian belief that sexual anxiety or learned fear of sex is behind an individual's sexual dysfunctions. That's why Hartman and Fithian, Masters and Johnson, and other behaviorally oriented sex therapists emphasized relaxation—to diminish or dispel an individual's fear of sex so the flow of sexual energy can resume its "natural" course. Hartman and Fithian also shared Master and Johnson's definition of male and female sexual success. Both measured the male's success by his capacity to penetrate a vagina with his penis and maintain his erection long enough to bring his female partner to orgasm, and both, in turn, measured the female's success by her capacity to be penetrated by a penis and experience an orgasm from its thrusting.

The most glaring difference between the Masters–Johnson and Hartman–Fithian approaches to sex therapy was the way Hartman–Fithian focused on a woman's body, particularly her vagina, which they referred to as "the organ of accommodation."[6] For them, when conducting sex therapy, the first order of business was to determine whether a woman has "any sensation or awareness in the vagina."[7] Thus, during the first days of treatment, Hartman and Fithian asked their women patients to focus on the feelings in their vagina, with the therapist's examining fingers inside:

> We find that often nothing has ever been in the vagina long enough for her to have developed any perception, and that because of this, she may describe any movement as pain. This is easily determined if the pain is inconsistent in location. Both of us spend time stimulating the vaginal area to develop a more comfortable and relaxed feeling with something in the vagina.[8]

Hartman and Fithian were also convinced of the benefits of getting the husband more involved in his wife's vagina, which may explain why, during the first week of treatment, they asked him to insert into his wife's vagina a plastic speculum that had a flashlight attachment:

> This allows him to look into the vagina and see the vaginal walls and the cervix and its opening, and he is able to see the area that has been forbidden for so long in our culture.... It helps him become comfortable with the vagina, and touching the genital area. Some men are very apprehensive about any genital contact with their partner. Their participation helps work through their fears in a situation where they can be helped.[9]

This strategy for demystifying the vagina accords with Hartman and Fithian's belief that a vagina is part of a muscular system that requires regular maintenance and exercise, in contrast to a penis, which, they believed, requires no maintenance or exercise apart from routine copulation. Accordingly, they exhorted women patients to tone up their vaginas in a series of exercises designed to make that organ tighter and more responsive to penetrative sex,[10] a modification that they believed should enhance not only a woman's pleasure but her male partner's as well.

> If the vaginal vault is loose, the penis going in and out of the vagina may have little friction on the walls. We encounter males who lose their erection during intercourse because of this problem. Some women have asked their partner if they are in, which has been in the past considered a put down of the male, and has been defined as the cause of some impotence problems for their partner. Actually the woman was probably not feeling anything herself, and was not sure whether he was in or out due to an unconditioned muscle with no perception or because the vagina was loose and gaping, and there was no friction.[11]

Hartman and Fithian's sex therapy program followed the central precepts of the intercourse imperative—for example, sex is natural, everyone is sexual, sex equals intercourse, women's consent is assumed, and women can and should coordinate their sexual responses to men's. But it was also anathema to scientific, university-sponsored behavioral research.[12] Hartman and Fithian claimed extensive laboratory research on non-orgasmic women, but never published their findings.[13] Their book, *Treatment of Sexual Dysfunction* (1972), while highly influential among clinicians during the 1970s and early 1980s,[14] was also largely ignored by sex therapy scholars. By contrast, university-sponsored behavioral sex therapy research, led by Temple University's Joseph Wolpe, was widely published and cited, with Wolpe's, *Psychotherapy by Reciprocal Inhibition* (1958) and *The Practice of Behavior Therapy* (1968), receiving as many academic citations as Masters and Johnson's international best-sellers, *Human Sexual Response* and *Human Sexual Inadequacy*.

Systematic Desensitization

Wolpe's most important contribution to sex therapy is a behavior modification technique called "systematic desensitization"—the "progressive weakening of a habit through repeated nonreinforcement of the responses that manifest it," a technique he originally developed in the 1950s in laboratory studies with cats.[15] Wolpe gave cats a series of electric shocks while they fed in their box, with the result that the cats soon refused to eat in that location, a behavior that persisted long after the shocks had been suspended and despite extended periods of food deprivation. Wolpe sought to reverse the cats' refusal to eat in their box by moving the cats and their box to a room that bore little resemblance to the room where they had been shocked. As Wolpe expected, the cats easily learned to eat in the new room. Next, he offered them food in a room that bore a slightly closer resemblance to the room where they had been shocked, and, as before, the cats easily learned to eat in that room. Continuing the desensitization pattern, he offered food to the cats in a room that bore a still closer resemblance to the room where they had been shocked, until, gradually, step by step, the cats were able to feed in the original room where they had been shocked.

In 1963, Arnold A. Lazarus extended Wolpe's systematic desensitization technique to women's sexual disinterest. First, he taught his women patients, whom he described as "frigid," to isolate the various muscle groups in their bodies, from their forehead, face, and so on, down to their toes, and then to "let go" of the tension in each muscle group. Second, he asked them to draw up a list of sexual situations that aroused fear, ranking them from strongest to weakest. Then he asked them to relax their muscles while they imagined the weakest fear-arousing sexual situation on their list. Once they could imagine that situation without their usual fear response, they were asked to imagine the next fear-arousing situation on the list, again, in a state of total relaxation. This process was then repeated with each fear-arousing sexual situation, moving up gradually, from one fear-arousing situation to the next, until they could imagine all the situations on their list without experiencing fear.[16]

To clarify how this technique works, Lazarus provided the case example of Mrs. A, aged twenty-four, who had been married two and a half years but had had intercourse less than two dozen times. She said she sometimes enjoyed hugging and kissing, but found intercourse painful and felt "disgust and anxiety at the whole messy business."[17] While Lazarus claimed that Mrs. A "sought treatment of her own accord,"[18] it is important to note that he never clarified what he or Mrs. A meant by this, a significant omission in light of Lazarus's report that Mrs. A decided to begin therapy because of her suspicion "that her husband had developed an extramarital relationship."[19] All of this suggests that, rather than beginning therapy "on her own accord," Mrs. A. may have been pushed into it by unfavorable marital circumstances. She may have felt that unless she became more successful at meeting her husband's sexual needs, he would leave her for another woman, an interpretation supported by her husband's fruitless efforts to increase his wife's interest in sex by providing her with books on sexual topics and techniques.[20] Although she obligingly read everything he gave her, he remained frustrated since the books had left her cold, an example of what Foucault called "the rule of lateral effects," whereby a so-called sexual dysfunction has its most intense effects on those who do not have the dysfunction.[21] This can also be seen as an example of reciprocal causality,[22] whereby a male partner's distress over his female partner's low sexual desire adds to her own distress, a pattern consistent with the finding that women diagnosed with low sexual desire who have a male partner are much more likely to feel distressed about their sexual functioning than are single women.[23]

The question of Mrs. A's motivation is important because an individual who enters into behavioral sex therapy showing no clear interest in sex except, perhaps, as a means to achieve some other end, such as saving her marriage and making her husband happy, does not fit a behavioral model specifically designed to extinguish sexual fears and anxieties. A woman is a candidate for behavioral sex therapy, according to Wolpe and Lazarus, when her sexual disinterest is related to fears or anxieties about sex, since those negative reactions can be extinguished by relaxation techniques. But if her sexual disinterest bears no relation to fears or anxieties, if her disinterest is simply inborn, she is not treatable. Wolpe cautioned,

> Occasionally, one encounters a woman whose sexual response system seems somehow to have failed to develop. She does not recall ever having known sexual arousal and gives no history of distressing sexual experiences that might have led to conditioned inhibition. It must be supposed that her deficiency is constitutional, and *there seems to be no available solution to the problem.*[24]

To restate Wolpe's caution in a slightly different way, a therapist cannot create or implant sexual desire in a woman, or in anyone else,[25] a position that is fundamentally the same as Masters and Johnson's. A therapist can only hope to eliminate or reduce the fears and anxieties that inhibit an individual's constitutional capacity for sexual arousal. The problem with this admonishment, as evidenced by Lazarus's management of Mrs. A's sexual disinterest, is that sex therapists hardly ever take it seriously. Lazarus does not mention the possibility that Mrs. A had a constitutional disinterest in sexual activity, a critical omission in light of the intransigence of that kind of inhibition: When a constitutional sexual inhibition occurs, Wolpe counseled, "I know of nothing that can be done about it. Perhaps one day we shall have ways of making people like things that they do not like, but we do not have them now."[26]

Was Lazarus attempting to make Mrs. A like something she did not like? The case study reveals only that Lazarus did not explore the issue in determining her treatment. Equally important, the case study does not explore the possibility that Mrs. A's sexual disinterest is person- and/or behavior-specific. Mrs. A may have found her husband sexually appealing at some point, but at the time she began therapy, she did not. She may or may not have had any specific complaints about her husband. None of that information was included in the case study. Mrs. A did, however, make it clear that, sexually, her husband turned her off. If Lazarus had asked Mrs. A about her relationship with her husband to see if he was doing something that elicited a negative sexual response, and she said yes—if she was able to identify a behavior (or behaviors) that dampened her sexual interest in him—then, perhaps, her husband could also be encouraged to change his displeasing behavior to accommodate his wife. As a hypothetical, say Mrs. A shared that when her husband attempted to have sex with her, all she could think about was the fact that he smelled like a sewer. If that information was obtained and shared with Mr. A, perhaps he would decide to take a bath before he made his next sexual advance, and, then, hopefully, Mrs. A would not feel as much "disgust and anxiety at the whole messy business." According to the case record, however, Lazarus did not pursue this line of inquiry. Instead, he plunged ahead with Mrs. A's systematic desensitization, asking her to draw up a list of sexual situations that aroused fear in her, with the most disturbing items at the top of the list:

1. Having intercourse in the nude while sitting on husband's lap.
2. Changing positions during intercourse.
3. Having coitus in the nude in a dining room or living room.
4. Having intercourse in the nude on top of the bed.
5. Having intercourse in the nude under the bed covers.
6. Manual stimulation of the clitoris.
7. Husband's fingers being inserted into the vagina during precoital love play.
8. Caressing husband's genitals.
9. Oral stimulation of the breasts.
10. Naked breasts being caressed.
11. Breasts being caressed while fully clothed.
12. Embracing while semi-clothed, being aware of husband's erection and his desire for sex.
13. Contact of tongues while kissing.
14. Having buttocks and thighs caressed.
15. Shoulders and back being caressed.
16. Husband caresses hair and face.
17. Husband kisses neck and ears.
18. Sitting on husband's lap, both fully dressed.
19. Being kissed on lips.
20. Being kissed on cheeks and forehead.
21. Dancing with and embracing husband while both fully clothed.[27]

For a period of three months, three sessions per week, Mrs. A attempted to imagine each item on this list while in a state of total relaxation. She began with "Dancing with and embracing husband while both fully clothed" and ended with "Having intercourse in the nude while sitting on husband's lap," a procedure that, as far as Lazarus was concerned, had an extremely positive outcome:

> When item 7 on the hierarchy had been successfully visualized, Mrs. A "seduced" her husband one evening and found the entire episode "disgustingly pleasant." Thereafter, progress was extremely rapid, although the first two items were slightly troublesome and each required over 20 presentations before the criterion (a 30 second exposure without signaling) was reached. A year later Mr. and Mrs. A both said that the results of therapy had remained "spectacularly effective."[28]

The problem with Lazarus' assessment of Mrs. A's progress is the same problem he had in assessing Mrs. A's motivation for treatment and the same problem Freud had in assessing Dora's accounts of her sexual experience: a failure to value and seek out the details of her testimony. Judging by his case description, he asked no follow-up questions regarding what made Mrs. A's seduction of her husband "disgustingly pleasant," nor did he ask why she claimed that the results of therapy were "spectacularly effective." Without detailed answers to these questions, Lazarus (and his readers), could only guess at the meaning of these terms and the overall effect of Mrs. A's treatment. Did she find sex therapy "spectacularly effective" because, as a result, she could now experience sexual pleasure without any inhibitory fear? Or did she find sex therapy "spectacularly effective" because it helped her tolerate an act—much as ether had once helped a Victorian wife tolerate painful copulation—that she continued to dislike in the most fundamental ways but that was, nonetheless, necessary to her husband's happiness and to the preservation of her marriage? Was treatment so effective because it facilitated Mrs. A's sexual pleasure or because it facilitated her husband's? Was Mrs. A the chief beneficiary of her own deconditioning? Or was her husband the chief beneficiary of a treatment program that transformed his wife into a more serviceable sexual partner?

These sorts of questions rarely arise in the treatment of heterosexual men's sexual dysfunctions, but for different reasons. When women are in treatment for a sexual dysfunction, it is usually assumed that they want to change in a way that matches their spouse's sexual expectations. Therapists usually assume that a female patient wants what her male partner wants, and that the main goal is to achieve synchrony between them. But when males are in treatment for a sexual dysfunction, the most common therapeutic concern is how to help them perform intercourse in a way that matches their *own* expectations. Their own pleasure is what matters. Consider, for example, the three case studies of male "impotence" that Wolpe included in his first text on behavioral treatment. In none of the three was the wife or female partner's reaction to the man's sexual dysfunction factored into the case study. In the first, Wolpe noted that, on the man's wedding night, his patient "had not had his usual erection, and even when intercourse was imminent his erection was poor and became even worse after he had rushed out of bed to get a condom. Ejaculation occurred the moment his penis came into contact with the vulva."[29] While Wolpe did not include the wife's response, he did go into detail about the man's assessment of his problem, noting that "he was greatly embarrassed, slept poorly, and the next day felt very low. He was very worried at what happened and made no further attempt at intercourse for two days. At his next attempt, he again failed to get a satisfactory erection and again ejaculated very prematurely, becoming as a result even more alarmed."[30]

As the previous passage illustrates, what receives the greatest share of therapeutic attention is the man's own assessment of his sexual dysfunction. This should be compared to the treatment of a woman's sexual dysfunction, where her male partner's assessment is often given as much (or more) importance as the woman's. Accordingly, Lazarus documented the success of Mrs. A's treatment by noting that "a year later Mr. and Mrs. A *both* said that the results were spectacularly successful" (emphasis added).

To understand the difference between the way sex therapy is organized for men and the way it is organized for women, it might prove helpful to examine Wolpe's instructions to men seeking treatment for their sexual dysfunction, in particular, how these instructions were geared to helping men feel comfortable performing the sex acts they want to perform, at the pace comfortable for them:

> The patient is told to inform his sexual partner (quoting the therapist if necessary) that his sexual difficulties are due to absurd but automatic fears in the sexual situation, and that he will overcome them if she will help him, i.e., if she will participate on a few occasions in situations of great sexual closeness without expecting intercourse or exerting pressure toward it. He is to ask her to be patient and affectionate and not to criticize. Assured of her cooperation, he is to lie in bed with her in the nude in a perfectly easy, relaxed way, and thereafter to do just what he really feels like doing *and no more*. He has no duty at any stage to reach any criterion of performance.[31]

Now try imagining these same instructions being given to Mrs. A. Could Mrs. A have informed her husband that her sexual difficulties are "due to absurd but automatic fears"? If Mrs. A had, what absurd fears would she describe? Could she have told her husband that she finds intercourse painful, disgusting, and messy? Are those fears? Or are they descriptions of her honest, unfiltered reactions to intercourse? If she really found intercourse painful, disgusting and messy, as she told Lazarus, then, of course, the idea of performing that act would arouse fear in her, as would the prospect of performing any other act that she found painful, messy, and disgusting. In that case, however, the fear of performing those acts would not precede her negative reactions; the negative reactions would come first, producing fear of performing them as an effect. While Mrs. A probably could have told her husband to lie in bed in the nude with her in a perfectly relaxed way, and he, given his interest in sex, would have likely agreed, the problem is that Mrs. A had no interest in lying naked with him in the first place. To the contrary, embracing him in bed while semi-nude was the twelfth most fear-arousing sex situation on her list of twenty-one, and having her naked breasts caressed figured as her tenth most fear-arousing situation. The critical point is that Mrs. A's negative reactions to sex were not necessarily the result of inhibitory conditioning; they were not necessarily the result of fear or anxiety. And absent any detailed inquiry into the genesis of these negative reactions and the meaning they had for her, Mrs. A's "spectacularly successful" treatment may have achieved something quite different than Lazarus imagined. It is possible that Mrs. A, through systematic desensitization, learned to tolerate an unpleasant and painful procedure—intercourse—which she believed she needed to tolerate, because her husband demanded that procedure as a precondition for continuing their marriage. If that's true, then for Mrs. A and her husband, therapy may have indeed succeeded "spectacularly," but in completely different ways.

Behavioral sex therapists generally do not explore the genesis of a woman patient's limited interest in intercourse, perhaps because they regard women as unreliable reporters of their own sexual experience. Even Wolpe—the therapist-scientist who invented systematic desensitization and subsequently forewarned therapists that women's disinterest in sex can sometimes be constitutional and therefore untreatable—paid relatively little heed to the origins of his female patients' sexual reticence. Consider this example of how he treated a woman "who had for years had a very good sexual relationship with her husband" but sought treatment when, as a result of escalating discomfort, she could no longer tolerate copulating with him. Wolpe's comments about the genesis of her problem only reference her husband's desire to insert his penis into her vagina, but say nothing about her own sexual motivations, nothing, that is, beyond cataloguing her wish to please her husband: "Because of her great affection for her husband, she had gone on permitting intercourse; but it was so aversive that she had become completely frigid, with marked vaginismus. Even after the vaginismus had been treated and intercourse was no longer painful, the vaginismus persisted so that it was impossible for her husband to gain entry."[32] This is how Wolpe described her treatment:

I instructed the patient to relax and to imagine, at first, a very thin rod (about 1/8 in. in diameter) being inserted a depth of ½ in. into her vagina. This produced anxiety. I continued repeating the scene until the anxiety disappeared. I then gradually increased the length of the rod's insertion, and subsequently repeated the sequence with progressively wider rods. When the width of the *imaginary* rod had reached ½ in., I arranged for the construction of a set of wax rods (bougies) that varied in diameter from 1/8 in. to 1½ in., that the patient was to use at home, starting with the insertion of the 1/8 in. bougie into her vagina, slowly, inch by inch. Thereafter, *in vivo* "shadowing" a few widths behind the imaginary was continued. When we reached ¾ in. diameter in imagination, movement such as would occur during coitus was introduced. This was a new source of anxiety which required repeated scene presentations for its desensitization. Then, movement with the bougie was started. Increasingly rapid movement came to be comfortably tolerated. At this point, I began to encourage careful experimentation with actual coitus, which became possible very soon, without producing vaginismus or any anxiety.[33]

Wolpe's technique, and this example, are quite famous, but as I read and reread Wolpe's description of how the treatment proceeded, I could not help thinking about the woman, his patient, whose significance as a human appears to have been reduced to that of a receptacle capable of receiving a series of imaginary and real rod-shaped objects into her vagina, culminating in the reception of her husband's penis. Wolpe described the case as a success because, like many of the others described in the sex therapy literature, the woman patient, in the end, was able to accept a penis into her vagina. But the question remains, why did Wolpe exclude any information on her motivation and frame of mind? Why did he see the intercourse goal as so important that it justified portraying her simply as an orifice that needed to learn to accept increasingly large objects until, finally, that orifice could comfortably accommodate a penis?

Wolpe was not alone. In Wolpe's day, and for many years after, this is how women diagnosed with vaginismus were treated. It was the norm. To illustrate, consider these homework instructions for women suffering from vaginismus who were receiving treatment at the Forest Hospital Sexual Dysfunction Clinic, in Des Plaines, Illinois, during the early 1970s.[34]

1. Proceed to inserting of the dilators by the husband with no direction from his wife.
2. After this has been accomplished several times, the wife ends each session by gently moving the last dilator back and forth a number of times before removing it (simulating intercourse).

3. After this step is successful, the husband's hand moves the last dilator back and forth with the wife's hand controlling it. Success here is followed by the husband supplying the control.
4. After this, successful intercourse is accomplished by the strict adherence to the following instructions:
   a. The husband lies on his back.
   b. The wife squats above him.
   c. Much lubrication is used on the erect penis and around the outside of the vagina.
   d. The woman gently puts her vagina around the penis, the man remaining motionless. After the vagina is completely around the penis, the woman stays motionless and experiences her "quiet vagina" surrounding the erect penis. She then slowly moves the vagina up and down the shaft of the penis, stopping at any development of pain or fear of pain. This exercise is repeated on at least a dozen future occasions before intercourse is attempted in any other position.

Manual stimulation of the clitoris to orgasm is recommended during the last few of these dozen sessions.[35]

The Intercourse Imperative

For behavioral sex therapists, as far as intercourse is concerned, the matter of a woman's feelings, motivations, consent, or lack of consent appears as a minor consideration, as Wolpe and Lazarus and the next case example demonstrate. In these representative cases from the 1960s and 1970s, sex therapy valued intercourse for women partnered with men, not for the manner in which it is accomplished, nor for what it means to the women who engage in it. What mattered more is that intercourse simply occurs, with orgasm resulting for at least one of the participants.[36] The rightness and naturalness of intercourse operated as a kind of unstated, foundational principle of how to address heterosexual women's sexual dysfunctions, which may explain why, in all behavioral case studies demonstrating systematic desensitization for heterosexual women, the hierarchy of sexual fears always ends with sexual intercourse.

Following are two examples of a "typical hierarchy of scenes" for desensitizing women's sexual anxiety. The first is from an article published in the journal of *Behavior Research and Therapy* in 1966, and the second is from an article published thirty-one years later, in the *Scandinavian Journal of Behaviour Therapy*. Both these hierarchies situate coitus or intercourse for a woman as the endpoint of her treatment. In both hierarchies, once the woman has succeeded in imagining scenes involving intercourse without exhibiting signs of fear or anxiety, the desensitization procedure and her treatment are over. Neither article explains why the hierarchy ends with coitus. The importance of intercourse is simply taken for granted. While the first list purportedly addresses the problem of "frigidity" and the second addresses "vaginismus," and both lists begin at very different points and encompass very different scenes, both lists end at almost the same point, with penis–vagina intercourse. The first list concludes, simply, with "continuing coitus" while the second concludes with "enjoying coitus." How "enjoying" something can be imagined as a fear-provoking scene may seem oxymoronic, but the point remains the same. For both, coitus represents the apotheosis of a woman's sexual health.

Typical Hierarchy of Anxiety-Provoking Sex Scenes

1. Being kissed on the lips by husband
2. Same as above but with tongue contact
3. Breasts fondled while fully clothed
4. Undressing with husband in bedroom
5. Being kissed on lips while nude
6. Seeing husband with erection
7. Fondling breasts while nude
8. Mouth contact with breasts by husband
9. Nude in bed with husband preparatory to coitus
10. As above with initial body contact
11. As above with kissing on lips and breast fondling
12. As above immediately before intromission
13. Intromission
14. Continuing coitus (ventral-ventral)[37]

Typical Hierarchy of Anxiety-Provoking Sex Scenes

1. Contracting and relaxing the muscles of the pelvic floor in everyday situations.
2. Touching with a finger vulva and the outside of the labiae minora.
3. Touching with a finger the inside of the labiae minora; periferically.
4. Touching with a finger the inside of the labiae minora; closer to the introitus.
5. Moving the finger around everywhere in the vestibulum.
6. Finger towards the introitus.
7. Finger towards the introitus and open the vagina.
8. Finger slowly enter the vagina and slowly withdraw from it.
9. Finger moving around in the vagina. Withdrawing from and re-entering the vagina.

10. Gently pressing on the backwall of the vagina, so that it sinks downwards, i.e. opening the vagina even more than needed for one finger.
11. Creating an as clear a picture as possible of what happens when the vagina opens for one finger.
12. Two fingers towards the introitus.
13. Two fingers towards the introitus and open the vagina.
14. Two fingers slowly enter the vagina and slowly withdraw from it.
15. Two fingers moving around in the vagina and specially withdrawing the fingers.
16. Gently pressing the backwall of the vagina, so that it sinks downwards, i.e. opening the vagina even more than needed for two fingers.
17. Creating an as clear a picture as possible of what happens when the vagina opens for two fingers.
18. Steps (2–5 if necessary) 6–11 with one finger of the partner.
19. Steps 12–17 with two fingers of the partner.
20. Erected penis touching everywhere in the vestibulum.
21. Erected penis moving around everywhere in the vestibulum
22. Erected penis toward the introitus.
23. Erected penis towards the introitus and opening the vagina.
24. Penis slowly entering and slowly withdrawing from the outermost part of the vagina.
25. Penis entering more and more of the vagina's length.
26. Penis entering and withdrawing quicker.
27. Penis moving around in the vagina.
28. Penis thrusting.
29. Allowing ejaculation in the vagina.
30. Integrating the ability to perform coitus "in a technical way" into sexual interaction with the partner.
31. Maintaining arousal during coitus.
32. Enjoying coitus.[38]

When Sex Therapists Prescribe Intercourse

When sex therapists regard intercourse as the natural endpoint for a woman's sex therapy, a goal so self-evident and necessary that it requires no defense or explanation, they might in some circumstances feel justified in forcing a woman to engage in intercourse. This appears to be the case in the following report, "An Innovation in the 'Behavioural' Treatment of a Case of Non-consummation due to Vaginismus," which appeared in the *British Journal of Psychiatry* in 1969. The case features a woman patient who sought psychiatric help because she could not tolerate intercourse.[39] While she and her husband often managed to bring each other to orgasm manually, they had never succeeded in "consummating" their marriage, that is to say, the husband never succeeded in ejaculating into his wife's vagina. Following each failed attempt, the patient would blame herself, and tearfully apologize. The husband, for his part, would commiserate with his wife's "dreadful pain," say that he would never do anything to purposefully hurt her, and discontinue the attempted coitus.

Their sex therapist was unsympathetic to the woman's alleged pain. As he saw it, the husband's commiseration and lack of follow-through were both unwarranted and harmful because they reinforced the resistance that characterized the wife's sexual dysfunction. Thus, he concluded that the couple's inability to consummate their marriage "had probably been maintained and consolidated by the submissive and sexually compliant attitudes of the patient's spouse."[40] Accordingly, the therapist focused on undoing this negative conditioning by teaching his patient to relax as she inserted progressively larger dilators into her vagina. The goal was to have her associate a positive stimulus—her relaxed state—with having something in her vagina that had the approximate size and shape of a penis. He reasoned that this should give her "confidence about the obvious adequacy (for coitus) of her vagina and dispel any fears that she might be 'torn inside' by the male organ."[41]

After six sessions, the wife claimed that she had grown accustomed to keeping the largest dilator in her vagina; she said that it was no longer disturbing, and she now felt ready to attempt intercourse. The therapist then asked her to tell her husband to prepare to engage in protracted love-play, during which he should do everything in his power to fully rouse her to an affectively charged physical receptivity and response. In addition, the therapist asked her to tell her husband "to ignore any protests of discomfort from her, since as he continued to stimulate her and to proceed with coitus she would become fully roused and relatively insensitive to pain, which would dissolve into pleasure culminating in orgasm."[42]

Four weeks later, the patient reported that after many attempts at intercourse and her husband's complete cooperation, penetration had still not been accomplished. It was simply too difficult. Every time he attempted to insert his penis into her vagina, she reacted with spasms and pain, and, as a consequence, he felt he had to discontinue. Again, he could not tolerate the idea of hurting her.

The therapist, on hearing this account, invited the husband and wife to see him together, at which time he told the husband that "he was over-sensitive to his wife's discomfiture and, by 'colluding' with her not to proceed with coitus when she gave minimal cues of pain, was partly responsible for the failure of therapy."[43] The therapist's use of the word "colluding," in this context, suggests that the husband and wife had entered into something akin to criminal conspiracy to avoid the wife's natural obligation to copulate. Applying the term *colluding* to describe a husband's overly solicitous behavior—his refusal to force penetration despite his wife's resistance—is not unique to this case. As recently as 1999, in an article appearing in the *Journal of Nervous & Mental Diseases*, the authors of "Does Vaginismus Exist? A Critical Review of the Literature" claimed that the most common explanation for vaginismus accepted by psychiatrists, gynecologists, and other sex therapists "is that the male partner has been chosen because he is passive and unassertive, and the couple is involved in an unconscious *collusion* to avoid intercourse."[44]

In this case study, after the sex therapist accused the husband of "colluding" with his wife to avoid intercourse, he told him, by way of encouragement,

> that full sexual arousal and orgasm were incompatible with pain, which would diminish reciprocally as his wife became more excited; *that he should ignore any complaints of pain either overt or implied, since it would be necessary for him by persistent and skillfully aggressive techniques to overcome his wife's resistance to full intercourse.* . . . finally, he was advised that if a spasm should develop during penile penetration he should not withdraw, but should remain where he was until the spasm and associated pain disappeared, when he was to continue penetration in a leisurely and unhurried manner.[45]

The italicized portion of the therapist's advice suggests an acceptance of marital rape. The therapist was, after all, advising the husband to force intercourse by ignoring his wife's complaints and employing "persistent and skillfully aggressive techniques to overcome his wife's resistance to full intercourse." From the professional perspective of behavioral sex therapy, the therapist may have seen himself as simply treating a patient with a psychiatric disorder. Her avoidance of intercourse defined her as a sick person in need of help. The question of her pain, therefore, as well as her husband's sympathetic response, interfered with the couple's progress toward the goal of curing her vaginismus. This assessment has pervaded the field of sex therapy as a whole, as evidenced by the fact that, among the thirty-seven sex therapy practitioners and scholars who have cited this case report in academic journals and papers, none has mentioned rape or cruelty as a possible concern.[46]

After the joint session with the husband and wife, the wife finally managed to achieve "full penetration," and the couple succeeded in consummating their marriage. Ten months later, on follow-up, the therapist noted that the husband and wife were performing intercourse on a routine basis, "frequent and sustained (technically adequate) coitus (up to seven minutes) from which the wife derived pleasure," albeit, without "a sensation comparable to the climaxes she had enjoyed through clitoral stimulation."[47]

The "technically adequate" coitus that ensued may have cost the couple months of painful, often humiliating effort, and for the woman, whose transformation was at issue, it produced nothing comparable to the pleasure she had experienced through the type of sexual activity she enjoyed prior to treatment. Nonetheless, the psychiatrist labeled this accomplishment a "therapeutic success" because the goal of sustained and repeated vaginal intercourse was met. For Masters and Johnson, for behavioral sex therapists, and for sex therapists in general, the medical, therapeutic precedence of heterosexual intercourse represents an unquestioned assumption. No matter what couples prefer to do in bed, regardless of their pain or pleasure, orgasmic intercourse is the designated determinant of success.

PART 3
CONTEMPORARY SEX THERAPY

6
Doublethink

> To know and not to know . . . to hold simultaneously two opinions which cancelled out, knowing them to be contradictory and believing in both of them, to use logic against logic. . . . Even to understand the word "doublethink" involved the use of doublethink.
> —George Orwell, *1984*

The 1980 *Diagnostic and Statistical Manual of Mental Disorders* (*DSM-III*) was the first *DSM* specifically oriented to a research-based medical model.[1] In keeping with that new model, the American Psychiatric Association (APA) decided against listing homosexuality as a psychiatric disorder, since there is no research evidence that homosexual behavior is inherently distressful or maladaptive.[2] At the same time, the APA chose to categorize people who have little or no interest in sex as psychiatrically disordered in the very same *DSM*, despite the fact that, as with homosexuality, we have no research evidence that having little or no interest in sex is inherently distressful or maladaptive.

A second incongruity between the stated goals of the *DSM-III* and the handling of sexual disorders also concerns the question of distress. While the APA insisted that a psychological pattern, to qualify as a psychiatric disorder, must be inherently distressful to the person who has the pattern, and not merely distressful to the people they interact with,[3] when it came to specifying the diagnostic features of "inhibited sexual desire," the distress criterion was changed to read: "In actual practice this diagnosis will rarely be made unless lack of desire is a source of distress to *either* the individual or his or her partner."[4] With this modification, a woman does not need to feel distressed about her lack of interest in sex to be diagnosed with a sexual inhibition; it's enough that her partner/husband is distressed about it. The APA's motivation for empowering men in this way, and for treating sexual dysfunctions differently from other kinds of psychiatric disorders, is unclear. The APA did not acknowledge that it was operating with different standards, as it did not consider any problems that might arise from treating sexual dysfunctions differently from other kinds of psychiatric disorders. Robert L. Spitzer, the psychiatrist who led the task force charged with redoing the *DSM* in accordance with a research-based model, argued that only clearly defined psychiatric disorders ought to be in the *DSM-III*, as opposed to "all of the forms of human psychological development which are judged by the profession or some members of the profession as less than optimal."[5] Despite this commitment to evidence-based determinations of disorder, neither Spitzer, nor the APA, identified research showing that a woman's disinclination to copulate passed as a behavior indicative of mental illness. Instead, they focused on the "less than optimal" standard, crediting the partner's/husband's discomfort as sufficient for labeling lack of sexual discomfort pathological.

This chapter examines how psychiatry, and sex therapy, in general, survived with different, even contradictory standards for diagnosing and treating sexual dysfunctions, standards that were particularly disadvantageous to women. Psychiatry and sex therapy managed "to hold simultaneously two opinions which cancelled out" by denying, diverting, and dismissing information supporting the hypothesis that a woman's disinclination to copulate might simply be a normal behavior variant or a situationally specific by-product of her relationship with her (male) partner.

Motivational Context Not Needed

To begin, let's consider a case study published by the APA's *DSM-III Case Book: A Learning Companion to the Diagnostic and Statistical Manual* (1981). Next is the original case study in full.

> Mr. and Ms. B.
>
> Mr. and Ms. B. have been married for 14 years and have three children, ages 8 through 12. They are both bright and well educated. Both are from Scotland, from which they moved 10 years ago because of Mr. B.'s work as an industrial consultant. They present with the complaint that Ms. B. has been able to participate passively in sex "as a duty," but has never enjoyed it since they have been married.
>
> Before their marriage, although they had intercourse only twice, Ms. B. had been highly aroused by kissing and petting and felt she used her attractiveness to "seduce" her husband into marriage. She did, however, feel intense guilt about their two episodes of premarital intercourse; during their honeymoon, she began to think of sex as a chore that could not be pleasing. Although she periodically complied with intercourse, she had almost no spontaneous desire for sex. She never masturbated, had never reached orgasm, thought of all the variations such as oral sex as completely repulsive, and was preoccupied with a fantasy of how disapproving her family would be if she ever engaged in any of these activities.
>
> Ms. B. is almost totally certain that no woman she respects in any older generation has enjoyed sex, and that despite the "new vogue" of sexuality, only

sleazy, crude women let themselves act like "animals." These beliefs have led to a pattern of regular, but infrequent, sex that at best is accommodating and gives little or no pleasure to her or her husband. Whenever Mrs. B. comes close to having a feeling of sexual arousal, numerous negative thoughts come into her mind, such as "What am I, a tramp?" "If I like this, he'll just want it more often." Or "How could I look myself in the mirror after something like this?" These thoughts almost inevitably are accompanied by a cold feeling and an insensitivity to sensual pleasure. As a result, sex is invariably an unhappy experience. Almost any excuse, such as fatigue or being busy, is sufficient for her to rationalize avoiding sex.

Yet, intellectually, Ms. B. wonders, "Is something wrong with me?" She is seeking help to find out whether she is normal or not. Her husband, although extraordinarily tolerant of the situation, is in fact very unhappy about their sex life and is very hopeful that help may be forthcoming.[6]

This case study, originally published in 1981 as a part of a guide to the *DSM-III*, was reproduced, word for word, in the 1989 *DSM-III-R Case Book*, the 1994 *DSM-IV Case Book*, the 2002 *DSM-IV-TR Case Book*, and the fifth edition of Comer's *Abnormal Psychology* (2004). The study's importance for psychiatry and sex therapy is its demonstration that a clinician does not have to inquire into how disliking sex impairs a woman's mental or social functioning, nor does a clinician have to inquire about her subjective distress.[7] At the same time, while the case study showed that Ms. B. complied with her husband's desires "periodically" and "passively" as a "duty," these accommodations were not sufficient to earn her a clean bill of psychiatric health. She also had to enjoy the sex acts—she had to reciprocate her husband's pleasure and excitement. Since Ms. B. clearly did not, she was diagnosed with "inhibited sexual desire" and "inhibited sexual excitement," and was left, at the end of the case report, wondering if she was "normal."

The case study elides the question of Ms. B.'s motivations. Despite acknowledging that Ms. B. performed sexually for her husband "passively, as a 'duty,'" the authors did not consider in their report the possibility that Ms. B. had been performing under duress. And at no point did the authors consider that Ms. B.'s lack of interest in sex might have something to do with the way she and Mr. B. interact. The study's last sentence ("Her husband, although extraordinarily tolerant of the situation, is in fact very unhappy about their sex life and is very hopeful that help may be forthcoming"[8]) may suggest that Mr. B.'s "extraordinary" tolerance for his wife's perceived sexual failing had been wearing thin, but the authors did not consider whether or how Ms. B. had been affected by her husband's disappointment. Ms. B. was described as adamantly anti-sex, and Mr. B. as pro-sex, but the case study includes no discussion of how they managed their conflict, nor does it inquire into how power was exercised in their relationship. The motivational context of her alleged sexual inhibition was treated as irrelevant. As a result of these omissions, the case study, reproduced in the *DSM Case Book* and referenced in psychiatric texts for more than two decades, conveys the message that psychiatrists and other sex therapy professionals do not need to ask how a woman's husband or partner influences her sexuality.

The Language of Sensory Experience

In sex therapy, the language of sensory experience has historically been used to bypass discussion of a couple's relationship, including discussion of what the partners mean to each other and what sex means to them in this relationship. By focusing almost exclusively on sexual techniques and arousal, in the Masters and Johnson model, sex therapists could bypass the question of what individuals hope to get out of sex, how well their sexual experiences match their needs and expectations, and whether they feel in any way coerced. Such issues are at the heart of a case study, "Female Orgasmic Disorder" (Donahey, 2010), which appeared in the second edition of the *Handbook of Clinical Sexuality for Mental Health Professionals*. In the study, Laura, a patient in treatment for her alleged orgasmic deficiency, reportedly told her therapist that she "worries that she is letting [her husband] down because she is unable to orgasm."[9]

Laura's concern with "letting her husband down" raises a number of questions. What made Laura imagine she might be disappointing her husband when she failed to orgasm? Did he withdraw? Did he sulk? Did he blame her or call her names? How did he signal his unhappiness with her failure to orgasm? Additional questions include: How did Laura feel about disappointing him? What did his disappointment *mean* to her? Did she worry that she was a bad wife? Did she worry that her husband would find her undesirable? Did she empathize with his disappointment? It would also be helpful to understand the role her husband's disappointment, or Laura's belief that he might be disappointed, played in motivating her to begin sex therapy. Did she want to improve her capacity to orgasm for her own sexual pleasure, or did she want to improve her capacity to orgasm to affirm and celebrate her husband's sexual performance? Did she want orgasms for herself or for him?[10] Those questions, if they were asked, do not appear in the case study. Instead, the therapist focuses on the physical dimensions of Laura's sexual experience, the micro detail of her sexual technique and progress toward orgasm:

LAURA: Victor and I start kissing and begin to undress each other. We'll lay on the bed and keep kissing and touching. He gets aroused very quickly.
THERAPIST: What do you mean?
LAURA: He'll get an erection in about 5 minutes.

THERAPIST: Are you aroused?

LAURA: Yes, but not as much as him. We'll touch some more; Victor mostly touching me.

THERAPIST: Where?

LAURA: All over my body.

THERAPIST: Are there any parts of your body you particularly like to be touched?

LAURA: Yes, my back, neck, breasts.

THERAPIST: Does he touch your genitals?

LAURA: Yes. He'll do this until I'm lubricated, and then we start having intercourse. We have intercourse a long time usually, about 10 minutes, so that I can try to have an orgasm, but it never happens. I get tired, and a little sore, and so I tell him to go ahead and have an orgasm. He does, but feels bad that I didn't have one.

THERAPIST: What happens after he has an orgasm?

LAURA: We hold each other, usually fall asleep.

THERAPIST: How are you feeling?

LAURA: I feel frustrated that I didn't have an orgasm. I wonder what's wrong with me. I don't want Victor to think he's done something wrong.[11]

Laura's last comments are striking and significant. She said she is frustrated that she didn't have an orgasm, but she also said she wanted to protect her husband against feelings of inadequacy. As in the previous case, it is not clear whether her central concern about sex with her husband is her experience or his. Does she want to "cure" her orgasmic deficiency to improve her husband's sexual experience or to improve her own? Instead of pursuing this path of inquiry, the therapist asks more questions about Laura's sexual sensations and techniques. The therapist wondered, for instance, if Laura and her husband "have engaged in oral stimulation, and if so, for how long and under what circumstances?" and whether Laura's "husband ever stimulates her manually simply for pleasure rather than doing it until she is lubricated enough for intercourse."[12] These performance questions may well be productive in sex therapy. Often, however, they are the first, and sometimes, the only questions therapists are trained to ask, so that questions about what a woman wants for herself are routinely overlooked. Sex therapy's emphasis, as Peggy Kleinplatz (1998) observed, is with the physical side of sexual activity—what patients' bodies are doing:

> Sex therapists may state that the goal of treatment is to diminish the focus on performance, to eliminate spectatoring, and to enable clients to feel closer with their partners; yet, the actual techniques employed encourage clients to focus precisely on the externals and to turn off their own internal cues.[13]

Strategic Ignorance

Laura's case reveals that one way to sidestep conversation about a woman's sexual motivations, consent, and power relations is to stay focused on physical sensation, sexual technique, and arousal. Another way is to limit the number of questions that are asked, in which case, a therapist might accept as adequate whatever the patient or professional colleague has to say about the problem, showing relatively little interest in psychological and social/relational detail. Consider, for example, a case study from an article, "Sexual Desire/Arousal Disorders in Women" (Basson, 2006) appearing in the fourth edition of the *Principles and Practice of Sex Therapy*, a volume that the editor claimed "brings together the most current, evidence-based, clinically sophisticated, integrated and interdisciplinary approaches to the assessment and resolution of sexual complaints."[14] That case study began with this sentence: "Caroline, age 55 and 6 years post menopause, was referred because of low sexual desire—for some 8–10 years in her estimation, and for some 20 years according to her husband, George."[15] This sentence reveals that Caroline "was referred because of low sexual desire," but does not reveal what Caroline's "low sexual desire" meant to Caroline or how it was a problem for her. As the case study unfolded, her supposedly "low sexual desire" was neither defined nor explained. As published case studies collectively suggest, sex therapists often fail to question how the label "low sexual desire" applies to women; they appear to take its meaning for granted, as though some objective measure of "low sexual desire" is universally accepted and understood, like a universally accepted, objective measure of "low blood pressure." Basson, the author of the case study, later notes that "Caroline felt very abnormal, but on another level somewhat resentful given that she personally was content with no sex," but does not inquire what the term *abnormal* meant to Caroline or when or why she began feeling that way. Nor does the author pursue what Caroline was "somewhat resentful" about. Did she feel some one or some others had pushed her to have sex? Or that she'd been pushed into sex therapy? Did she feel her husband had pressured her in some way? Or that the referring physicians or counselors were imposing their belief that the absence of sexual desire is a serious problem? Alternatively, Caroline may have been expressing dissatisfaction with the absence of sexual feelings. If so, what was the nature of her dissatisfaction, and when did it begin?

We Simply Do Not Know

Fortunately, according to the case report, Caroline's sexual malaise, whatever its origins, whatever it represented, was cured almost immediately. As the therapist explained, after hearing that many women have close to zero spontaneous desire but go ahead anyway and engage in sex . . . Caroline totally changed her situation around between the first and second visit. We had suggested the couple might begin to discuss bringing back into their lives some nonintercourse sexual caressing and some "date like" contexts. However, no discussion occurred—just action.[16]

The "action" the therapist was referring to is the sexual activity that Caroline initiated with her husband: after her first session, she went home and, on two occasions, invited her husband to copulate with her.

What should be noticed here is that the therapist chose not to investigate how this apparent success had been accomplished, but "simply congratulated the couple" and told them to check back in six months, at which time the therapist reported that "their progress continued. . . . This truly appears to be an example of therapy that consisted solely of giving information."[17]

Here's the problem: if sex therapy success "consisted solely of giving information," what is the nature of this game-changing information? What information "totally changed her situation around between the first and second visit"? Is it that "many women have close to zero spontaneous desire but go ahead anyway and engage in sex?" Is it that a woman can and perhaps should consent to sex that she does not desire or want? A woman can go along with sex regardless of how she feels? If that is the information the therapist was alluding to, how could that have had such a dramatic impact on Caroline? Wouldn't she have already known, either from intuition or from her own experience, that a woman almost always has the option to go along with a man's demands for intercourse, whether or not she actually wants to have intercourse? Wouldn't she have already known that, unlike men, who require an erection, for women, wanting, desiring, or enjoying penetration is *not* a prerequisite for the accomplishment of penetration.[18] On the other hand, maybe Caroline didn't know that reluctant participation is regarded as normal.[19]

Today, despite the persistence of the intercourse imperative, the experience of unpleasurable, undesired, but consensual sex overlaps with many people's definition of coercive sex. To be sure, it can be difficult to isolate the element of coercion in sexual relationships, since coercion can range from physical threats and violence to something as seemingly innocuous as the perceived obligation to repay a spouse for doing the dishes.[20] At the same time, it is important to recognize that in the most recent national sample of women's experience of sexual violence in marriage (Basile, 2002), the question, "Have you ever had sex with a husband or intimate partner when you really did not want to?" served as the filter for sexual coercion against women.[21] That question, in other words, was the dividing line between women who have experienced some level of sexual coercion in marriage and those who have not. Accordingly, in that study, if women answered "yes," to that question, they were asked to specify the circumstances under which the unwanted sex occurred; among the seven possible answers, the second, "because you thought it was your duty to have sex with him when he wants to have sex,"[22] may have particular relevance to Caroline's treatment.[23] Caroline may have interpreted her therapist's statement that "many women have close to zero spontaneous desire but go ahead anyway and engage in sex" to be a directive to engage in intercourse regardless of her own preferences.

In her book, *Of Woman Born*, Adrienne Rich quoted a letter to Margaret Sanger (1928) in which a young woman represents this kind of sex as obligatory,

> I am not passionate, but try to treat the sexual embrace as I should, be natural and play the part, for you know it's so different a life from what girls expect.[24]

Caroline may have believed that her therapist wanted her to fake desire ("be natural and play the part") because that is what she, as a wife, owes her husband. As Adrienne Rich interpreted the letter to Sanger,

> the history of institutionalized motherhood and of institutionalized heterosexual relations (in this case, marriage), converge in these words from an ordinary woman of half a century ago, who sought only to fulfill the requirements of both institutions, "be natural and play the part"—that impossible contradiction demanded of women. What strategy handed from ashamed mother to daughter, what fear of losing love, home, desirability as a woman, taught her—taught us all—to fake orgasm?[25]

The strategy of faking orgasm handed down from "ashamed mother to daughter" is seemingly endorsed by Caroline's therapist. This may explain why this therapist declared immediate and total victory over her patient's sexual disinterest problem, thereby avoiding close inquiry into how that victory had been accomplished and what it might mean to Caroline. Had the therapist pursued this line of inquiry, she might have discovered that Caroline initiated intercourse as a gesture of capitulation, that Caroline consented to intercourse as an obedient subject rather than as an autonomous person. Indeed, if the therapist had asked Caroline why, after only one session, she adopted an entirely new, assertive approach to sex with her husband, the therapist might have learned that Caroline not only wanted to please him but wanted to please the therapist too. After all, the therapist had given every indication of wanting Caroline to become sexually active, not only by telling her that "many women have close to zero desire but go ahead anyway and engage in sex" but also by suggesting that Caroline and her husband should begin bringing back "sexual caressing" into their lives. Upon receiving this information, Caroline might have reasoned that the only way to win her therapist's approval, perhaps also the only way to avoid further pressure from her, was to give her the therapeutic win she so earnestly sought by forcing herself to engage in sexual activity she would have otherwise avoided. She might have decided, either consciously or unconsciously, to forfeit a portion of her personal autonomy in exchange for making others happy.

Granted, we commonly forfeit portions of our autonomy for others. We make the special run to the market, spend hours sitting through boring movies, and sometimes agree to look in on a friend's sick cat, not because we want to, but because it's important to someone we care about. It makes someone else feel better. Those kinds of behaviors are usually considered virtuous and tend to get catalogued under headings such as generosity, caring, and selflessness. However, it is also true that the people we care about can be too demanding and that we can forfeit too much for their benefit. And many have argued that forfeiting autonomy in the area of sexuality may represent a special case. According to Robin West, such forfeitures may be exceptionally costly to women's sense of selfhood. She identified four kinds of injury that women sustain from engaging in consensual but unwanted sex:[26] First, it injures women's capacity for self-assertion, since "acting on the basis of our own felt pleasures and pains is an important component of forging our own way in the world." Second, it injures women's sense of self-possession: "When we consent to undesired penetration of our physical bodies we have in a quite literal way constituted ourselves as . . . 'giving selves'—selves who cannot be violated because they have been defined as (and define themselves as) being 'for others.'" Third, it injures women's sense of autonomy: "When women consent to undesired and unpleasurable sex because of their felt or actual dependency upon a partner's affection or economic status . . . they have thereby neglected to take whatever steps would be requisite to achieving the self-sustenance necessary to their independence." Finally, it injures women's sense of personal integrity when they feel they have to lie about the reasons they engage in these unpleasurable and undesired sexual acts, when they feel compelled to say they enjoyed the whole thing.[27]

If Caroline's therapist had inquired into the sudden change in Caroline's sexual behavior, she might have discovered that Caroline initiated intercourse with her husband, not as a demonstration of personal empowerment, but as a demonstration of her damaged integrity and self-possession. On the other hand, when the therapist chose to remain ignorant of the reasons behind her patient's rapid shift of position, she had no chance of discovering whether Caroline had put on an act for others or of determining whether the price Caroline paid for accepting the intercourse imperative was her own authenticity. In the tradition of doublethink, the therapist may have chosen ignorance over knowledge. Rather than risk discovering the contradiction between female empowerment and the intercourse imperative, the therapist simply congratulated her patient on a job well done.

Women's Sexual Desire Is Complicated

Most women who are in therapy for low sexual desire do not experience instantaneous cures, either real or faked. This is partly because shifting from low desire to moderate or high desire for sex or for anything else is hardly ever easy. It's also because faking that kind of shift—in effect, sacrificing authenticity for conformity to a moral imperative—while doable, does not feel very good. As one heterosexual woman who participated in a study on the meaning of intercourse described her experience of having unwanted, albeit consensual, intercourse: "I came to feel like it was a great invasion.... Oh I could reach orgasm but it was very mechanical, you know. I mean you kind of 'if I do this then you do that, then I'll do this.' You know, very sort of boring."[28]

In sex therapy cases where women patients with low sexual desire seem to be having a hard time connecting with the kind of desire their male partners and therapists have in mind for them—cases where the patients are sometimes labeled resistant or difficult—their therapists may have a hard time too. They may have a hard time giving up their hope for a cure. Sex therapists may have a hard time suspending their foundational prejudice, even in the face of massive disconfirming evidence, that a woman's low sexual desire is a treatable disease. When such disconfirming evidence appears, instead of questioning the premise that low sexual desire is a medical/psychiatric problem, they may begin to question the adequacy of their knowledge and their skill as sex therapists. In other words, if sex therapists cannot cure heterosexual women of their disinclination to copulate, they may not then conclude that such a disinclination is normal, or constitutional, or that the hoped for cure does not exist; rather, they may conclude that the task of treating women's low sexual desire is uniquely challenging and that professional therapists should keep searching and experimenting until they have found the answers they are looking for.

This kind of doublethink response, which we might call "inattention to disconfirming evidence," has two main effects. On the one hand, sex therapy remains naïve to the problems and processes that comprise its female patients' most pressing concerns; on the other hand, that very naivete allows sex therapists to imagine themselves confronting real and complex, yet ultimately solvable puzzles. In the words of a sex therapist (Lief, 1995) who reluctantly gave up his efforts to cure his woman patient's low sexual desire only after her unexpected decision to discontinue treatment, "No clinical problem facing sex therapists is as complex and confusing as the diagnosis of hypoactive sexual desire disorder."[29] This claim is from an article, "Integrative Therapy in a Woman with Secondary Low Sex Drive," which appeared in a collection "intended to portray the 'nuts and bolts of clinical reality of sex therapy practice.'"[30]

The therapist, in this instance, was referring to a woman identified as Lil, a thirty-year-old mother of three. While the therapist said that Lil "had noted a gradual decrease in sexual desire," after the birth of her second child, he did not specify what brought her to sex therapy. Was she seeking to increase her sexual desire for herself, for her own pleasure, or for someone else's? As in Caroline's case, we simply do not know. The therapist, however, did go into considerable detail about the absence of Lil's sexual feelings, specifically, her lack of fantasies or sexual dreams, her failure to respond to sexual stimuli in books, movies, or television, and her claim that a sexual encounter with her husband feels like "an intrusion and invasion of her space." The therapist added that while Lil can become sexually aroused and orgasmic, it takes a lot of work, and any pleasure she gets out of it is insignificant compared to the costs.[31]

After describing Lil's experience of sex as veering between insignificantly pleasurable and significantly invasive, the therapist noted that "there is no pressure from her husband" to change. The therapist thus leaves unanswered any questions about the source of Lil's motivation to change. What made her *want* to want sex? The therapist's explanation is that Lil suffers from "an inner feeling that she is obligated to do this,"[32] suggesting that Lil's main problem is not her failure to enjoy sex, but rather her unshakeable belief that she should. In other words, Lil appears to suffer from a compulsion to perform sexual acts she does not enjoy, which suggests that she might have been better served by seeing a therapist who could help her extinguish this feeling of compulsion, as opposed to a therapist who, in labeling her sexual disinclination a psychiatric disorder, seemed to endorse that very compulsion. Lil might have been better served by seeing someone who could help her understand that it's normal and common to not enjoy sex—who could help her refrain from activities she doesn't enjoy— instead of a therapist whose goal is to unleash her untapped capacity for sexual desire, a capacity that neither she, nor anyone else, has demonstrated she actually has. According to the case study, Lil's therapist never mentioned this option. From the very first session, his singular purpose was to find a way to make Lil sexually responsive:

> I mentioned to her the various ways in which we could deal with this, from pharmacological treatment to psychological and I recommended that we try to work this out psychologically because the inhibition of desire and arousal seems to be related to the central theme of feeling that sex is an intrusion, an invasion of her space.[33]

Judging by the text, the therapist never considered that Lil's "feeling that sex is an intrusion, an invasion of space" does not have to be seen as a psychiatric disorder. In reporting Lil's case, the therapist does not consider why, in this day and age, when a lesbian woman can see a psychiatrist without risk of receiving a medical diagnosis and referral for sexual conversion treatment, heterosexual women should adhere to a different standard. His telling of Lil's therapy story doesn't examine the routine diagnosing of heterosexual women with a psychiatric dysfunction when they claim to dislike intercourse. As a result, Lil continued therapy for over a year, in a total of twenty-three sessions, during which time her therapist tried innumerable interventions in the hope of giving her a positive attitude toward sex. When one treatment intervention didn't work, instead of concluding that Lil's lack of sexual interest is constitutional and untreatable, the therapist reports simply shifting to a new treatment approach, and when that new approach didn't work, the therapist moved on to yet another approach, and so on, over and over, without declaring defeat until Lil withdrew from treatment. Thomas Kuhn called this the "puzzle-solving" model of "normal science," whereby scientists follow the prescripts and suppositions of an established paradigm, but never question the paradigm itself. Even though the predetermined paradigm may be nothing more than an untested, historical construct, Kuhn has observed that scientists treat it as the unquestioned basis from which their research proceeds.[34] In the case at hand, they have to defend the notion that a woman's low sexual desire is a curable disease, that women are inherently sexual whether they say they are or not, and that the ultimate expression of a woman's inherent sexual capacity is intercourse. While this model adjusts to signs of disconfirmation, like Ptolemy's model of the heavens, it doesn't stop to acknowledge the significance of those disconfirming signs. It keeps going, even in the face of empirical failure. After Lil's therapist had tried cognitive-behavioral approaches, including sensate focus and sensual massage exercises, after he tried "immersion therapy" whereby sexual desire is treated as a phobia, after he encouraged Lil to try to "bulldoze" her way through her sexual reticence by forcing herself to have sex, and after he tried pharmacological therapy, changing Lil's medication from Prozac to Wellbutrin and then injecting her with testosterone, all to no lasting effect, the therapist did not give up. Ignoring (or overlooking) the possibility that Lil's responses to sexual stimulation, while muted, may have been normal for her, the therapist decided to try yet another treatment approach on Lil. He decided that he and Lil might have better luck with Freudian psychoanalytic therapy.

As part of this approach, which spanned nine sessions, the therapist and Lil gained several insights into her family dynamics. For example, they came to see the connection between Lil's desire to leave home and her mother's oversolicitousness, they arrived at an understanding of the conflict between Lil's dependency on her mother and her wish to become an independent woman, they came to see Lil's perfectionism as a protest against her mother's disorganization, and they learned to regard Lil's need for space as a symptom of her fear of being engulfed, so that "by keeping sufficient distance from her husband she could maintain the fiction of being a fully autonomous person."[35]

Unfortunately, neither the therapist nor Lil had an opportunity to see if any of these insights had the desired effect on Lil's sexuality, because after the therapist pointed out these dynamics, Lil suddenly announced her desire to break off treatment. In keeping with Kuhn's model of "normal science" as "puzzle-solving," Lil's withdrawal from therapy did not cause the therapist to entertain the possibility that the standard sex therapy paradigm is wrong. Instead, he concluded that he and Lil might have been on the cusp of a therapeutic break-through; he imagined that he "had been too close to pay dirt and that was why she broke off treatment when she did."[36]

While the therapist's closing words reflect his disappointment and confusion at the way Lil's treatment ended, his confidence in the sex therapy paradigm remained unshaken:

> I was puzzled that deepening the patient's understanding did not seem to change much. I am also frustrated that here is a person who outwardly has everything going for her, an adoring successful husband, lovely children, more than enough money to be comfortable, some close caring friends, and in this one realm of her life she remains baffled, as baffled as I am that nothing seems to change the equilibrium. This is the hard part of therapy when you work hard and you have, from all appearances, a very cooperative patient, and nothing seems to work.[37]

The principal irony here is that, from the therapist's point of view, this patient had everything going for her ("an adoring husband, loving children"). Yet the therapist could only see her as a sad, tragically flawed figure, in desperate need of psychiatric help. So desperate was her need, according to her therapist, that no matter how many failures he experienced in treating her low sexual desire, no matter how frustrated he became, he could not give up the hope of giving Lil the one thing he was certain she needed for a happy, fulfilled life—a desire for sexual intercourse.

Prioritizing Sexual Coercion from an Earlier Time

At the close of the previous chapter, I suggested that any doubts that a British psychiatrist might have had about forcing a woman to engage in unwanted, painful intercourse may have been overridden by the psychiatrist telling himself that he was curing her vaginismus. She was a sick woman and she required treatment. The next case study reveals another sex therapy judgment that can similarly obscure the possibility that therapists are perhaps unwittingly endorsing sexual coercion: prioritizing sexual coercion from an earlier time over the sexual interactions—including coercion—that might be occurring in a woman's ongoing relationships.

In October 1989, the American Association of Marriage and Family Therapists held a conference in San Francisco during which a well-known sex therapist, Joseph LoPiccolo, interviewed a married couple with a chronic, seemingly intractable sexual discrepancy. The interview was conducted before a large audience of marriage and family therapists, and the American Association for Marriage and Family Therapy subsequently published the video of that session as part of a series of master therapist demonstrations.[38]

At the beginning of the session, the husband, aged forty-three, made it clear that if his wife, aged forty-one, did not become more sexually available and responsive, he would divorce her. "My wife doesn't like sex," he said. "I was going to get a divorce. She suggested counseling instead." When the wife was asked to explain the problem, she immediately blamed herself: "Sometimes I think it's probably me. A lot of times I thought it was physical or mental. A lot of it would be mental. Back when I was a child, a lot of things happened." She went on to say that she had been sexually abused by her stepfather and had flashbacks whenever she and her husband attempted to have sex. She said she had been in individual therapy for about two years to get over the trauma, but without success.

After the disclosure that she experienced flashbacks, the therapist devoted the next fifteen minutes, about one-quarter of the entire session, to questioning her about the abuse she sustained as a child. Among the therapist's questions, he asked, "How old were you when the abuse started?" "How often did this happen to you?" "What would actually happen when your stepfather molested you? Did he actually have intercourse with you?" "You can remember him coming up behind you and fondling your breasts, but can you remember him actually putting his penis inside your vagina?" "So you can remember him doing a lot of fondling of your breasts, and coming up behind you, [but] you can't remember if he actually had his penis in your vagina, or your anus, or your mouth, or if he made you touch his penis or he touched your genitals?" "If you were to guess, what would you think, did he actually have intercourse with you?" "Did he also ever physically assault you? Did he beat you?" The therapist addressed these and many other questions to the wife about the abuse, including questions about how much and for how long her mother knew, why her mother didn't try to protect her, whether her siblings were also abused, what her stepfather's motives might have been, and what she would like to tell him if he were still alive.

The wife was extremely cooperative. She tried to answer every question, but she struggled at times both because she could not recall details and because the details she could recall were so painful she broke into tears. "It was so awful, I can't remember." However, her tears and memory gaps did not appear to discourage the therapist. He continued to push for details on the abuse, one question immediately following the next, especially with regard to whether the stepfather had put his penis into her vagina ("If you were to guess, what would you think, did he actually?").

If sexual abuse represents a trauma in which a victim's power is taken away, the therapist, in introducing all these highly sensitive, sexual questions without first gaining his patient's permission, may have been inadvertently duplicating the abuse dynamic.[39] It's quite possible that the wife's capacity to give consent to (or to resist) this line of questioning might have been compromised by the therapist's professional authority, as well as by the fact that his questions were asked in front of a large audience of family therapy professionals who were strangers to her. To add to the unfairness, the therapist appeared to disregard the wife's complaints about her husband. Even though she said that she found her husband's sexual behavior inappropriate and excessive ("He is too interested in sex," she said. "It seems like that's the main thing in his life"), the therapist concentrated his attention on the husband's complaints about her.

In the therapist's defense, we should acknowledge that he may have been paying homage to Freud's early "chimney sweeping" technique, whereby patients are supposed to overcome repressed trauma by recovering painful memories, particularly those that originate in childhood and involve parent figures.[40] The therapist probably thought that recovering traumatic memories from the wife's distant past would do her good, a position that received a great deal of support during the 1990s with the ascendancy of trauma theory and books such as Caruth's *Trauma: Explorations in Memory* (1995) and Herman's *Trauma and Recovery: The Aftermath* (1992).

At the same time, by focusing on memories of the stepfather's abuse, the therapist may have erased any concern, or even awareness, that a woman who had been sexually coerced as a child may have been, and perhaps was still, a victim of sexual coercion in her marriage. Thus, the public discussion of one man's coercion—the stepfather's—could well serve as a cover for another's coercion, that of a husband who threatened to divorce his wife if she did not become more sexually available and responsive to him.

By dwelling on the sins of the stepfather, and in particular, by noting their effects on his victim, the therapist not only reached the conclusion that the wife's aversion to intercourse could be cured; he also formulated a plan for accomplishing the cure: the wife would have to undo what had been done to her. She would need to exorcise the abuse, sweep that trauma and its effects from her innermost being. It made no difference that she had been in individual therapy for years without success, or that she told the therapist she had no interest in having sex with her husband, or that the only reason she began treatment was to avoid divorce. The therapist was convinced that she would need to recall/relive her abuse in long-term individual therapy if she were to have any chance of becoming a member in good standing of the world of healthy, functioning sexual beings. Thus, the therapist told her that she would have "to go back and really work through what happened" to her. As he explained, "it's kind of like stepping on a nail. And you have a deep, deep puncture wound that goes in a couple of inches. On the surface, it's healed over. It's not even scabbed anymore. It's just a little red area on the skin. But down on the bottom, it's full of pus. It's infected. It's rotting flesh." The therapist then told her that her goal in therapy would be to "squeeze out all the pus, and clean out the wound from the bottom up, and heal it from the bottom up." He said that this approach would be very time-consuming, painful, and difficult ("You're bringing up a lot of very unhappy, very upsetting memories when you do that, and it will be necessary to do some work where you act as if your stepfather is still alive."), but it was also the only way her sexual problem could be treated.

Doublethink makes it possible that no one, not the therapist, not the husband, nor the wife, nor anyone in the audience, brought up the possibility that a woman who had been forced into sex as a child, was now, as an adult, being forced into a treatment program, the end goal of which—intercourse—was also unwanted and undesired. Ironically, the public denunciation of the stepfather's behavior may have even reinforced sex therapists' solidarity around the idea that sex, under ordinary circumstances, is positive and healthy—the case of the exception proving the rule.[41] As the therapist told the wife, "you missed out on one of the most physically pleasurable, emotionally rewarding, closest, warmest, nicest, most intimate parts of being a person, being a woman."

7
Men's Free Will

> I know this—a man got to do what he got to do.... On'y thing in the worl' I'm sure of, an' that's I'm sure nobody got a right to mess with a fella's life. He got to do it all hisself.
> —John Steinbeck, Grapes of Wrath (1939)

To better understand the gender asymmetry built into sex therapy, and more fundamentally, into Western culture, we should examine how sex therapy manages when it's a man who presents with the problem of low desire. Are the rules and expectations any different when it's the husband who wants less sex and the wife wants more? Does sex therapy treat husbands more respectfully, more empathically?

When a Man Feels Zero Desire

According to the case study, "Couple Therapy for Low Desire: A Systemic Approach" (Gehring, 2003), which originally appeared in the peer-reviewed *Journal of Sex and Marital Therapy*, Bill, a man nine years older than his wife Belle, had not shown any spontaneous sexual interest in her for the past year. That problem appeared to worsen the more Belle pressured him to perform.[1] However, in contrast to the way the problem of Caroline's low sexual desire had been described in the previous chapter, with the therapist suggesting she go home and become sexually active even if she "felt zero desire," Bill's therapist came to the conclusion after only one interview that there was nothing wrong with him. "It was not that Bill found Belle any less sexually attractive but that he had sexually shut down because of his present life situation."[2] According to the therapist, Bill was simply exhausted. He had to awaken each day at four in the morning so he could arrive at work at five and did not return home until six that evening. What made it even harder for Bill to get a good night's sleep, the therapist discovered, is that the couple slept in the same bed as their baby. Unlike Caroline's sexual disinterest, which was defined as a psychiatric issue, Bill's was not given a psychiatric diagnosis. Bill's therapist did not locate the problem inside Bill. Rather, the therapist externalized the problem, attributing Bill's sexual apathy to his living conditions. As the therapist explained, "His environment was not sexual for him with the baby present, so he remained neutral. And any spontaneous desire was infrequent in him because of his fatigue."[3] As a result of this interpretation, "Belle's anxiety that she was not attractive to Bill was reduced, and the couple was able to seek creative solutions, such as finding alternative space for their son's sleeping arrangement."[4] Unlike Caroline, who was sent home with the recommendation to go ahead and have sex with her spouse even if she didn't want to, Bill was prescribed no sexual activities or exercises. Moreover, the therapist, according to the case report, did not see any reason for follow-up visits to determine whether the frequency of intercourse had increased or decreased. In contrast to the way "low sexual desire" was managed for Caroline and other women, Bill was not required to change in any way to more successfully satisfy his spouse's sexual needs. The male patient's would-be sexual problem was defined out of existence, and, in fact, his female partner was the one "adjusted" by Bill's diagnosis and treatment; she was persuaded to become less anxious about her sexual attractiveness to Bill and therefore less likely demanding of his sexual performance.

A Wife Must Adapt

Susan–Nick

Another example of this gender asymmetry is the case of Nick, aged thirty-nine, a geologist, and his wife, Susan, aged thirty-three, a nurse, as described in an article, "Sexual Desire Disorders in Men" (Maurice, 2007), published in the *Principles and Practice of Sex Therapy*.[5] During Susan's earlier consultation with her family physician, she revealed that her husband was neither sexually active nor sexually motivated, a state of affairs she found extremely disturbing because, after nine years of marriage, she wanted children. The family physician then referred the couple to a psychiatrist, but Nick refused to continue after the first visit. Susan offered on several occasions to find another therapist, but Nick always balked. Finally, after Susan threatened to leave him, he consented to see a sex therapist. At their first meeting, Susan related that one of the things that first attracted her to Nick is that he did not immediately "pounce" on her like so many other men she had known. She went on to say that when they did have sex, she was the initiator and that shortly before their marriage, he began to refuse her sexual overtures. Now, she said, they rarely even touch one another and added that while she didn't want to lose Nick and enjoyed the life that they had built together, she felt she was "missing out" and was concerned that her "biological clock is ticking." Nick said his interest in sex was somewhere between negligible and nonexistent, an admission that prompted the therapist to give him a diagnosis of "lifelong/generalized hypoactive sexual desire disorder."

In contrast to the way the sex therapist approached Lil's sexual disinterest in the case examined in the previous chapter, Nick's therapist came to the immediate conclusion that there would be nothing to gain from attempting to treat Nick's sexual disinterest since he interpreted it as lifelong and constitutional. However, the therapist did not see this as a signal to give up on treating the couple altogether, but rather as a signal to shift the focus of treatment from Nick to his wife. The new goal consisted of helping Susan "adapt more successfully to what seemed minimally changeable, namely, Nick's level of sexual interest."[6] In other words, since the therapist assumed he couldn't increase Nick's level of desire, he figured he could at least try to decrease his wife's sexual expectations.

As part of the effort to lower Susan's sexual expectations, the therapist recommended that the couple go home and rather than practice sensate focus and other erotic exercises, the most common kinds of homework assignment when the female partner has little interest in sex, they were told to simply practice holding hands.[7] However, when they returned for their next therapy session, it became clear that minimal hand-holding had occurred between visits, largely as a result of Nick's lack of motivation. This led the therapist to suggest shifting the therapy focus away from touching entirely, focusing instead on the other parts of the couple's relationship. But this did not interest Nick, and, although Susan had threatened to leave him if he did not pursue therapy, the threat proved ineffectual. After only two more sessions, Susan phoned to say that her husband had decided to discontinue.

Dave–Alicia

According to the case of Dave and Alicia, as described in the article, "A Catalytic Approach to Sex Therapy" (Fraser and Solovey, 2004), published in *Quickies: The Handbook of Brief Sex Therapy*, after ten years of marriage, Dave seemed to have lost all interest in sex: "Alicia and Dave appeared for therapy with what they thought was an unusual problem—male frigidity."[8] While earlier in their marriage, Alicia said Dave's sexual appetite was "voracious," now the opposite was true. He had not initiated sex in six months, and when Alicia tried to interest him in sex, he made excuses and declined. At the initial interview, Dave reported that he was unsure whether he was still "in love" with Alicia and suggested that the more accurate term for his feelings would be "friendship." Moreover, the therapist noted that while Dave was "wondering what would happen if his feelings for her didn't return, he considered the possibility that he would leave the marriage."[9] The therapist also noted that Alicia had been working hard to get Dave sexually engaged again: "She had waited up for him when he was late for work, arranged candle-light dinners, worn sexy lingerie to bed, given him suggestive kisses, and asked him about what he was thinking and feeling about her. When he'd failed to respond in an assuring manner, Alicia had become tearful."[10]

The therapist hypothesized that there was an inverse relationship between Alicia's efforts to make herself sexually appealing to Dave and Dave's level of sexual interest. The harder she tried, the more he withdrew, and, as far as the therapist could see, by the time they began therapy, this cycle had become a preoccupation for Alicia; she was "spending most of her day dwelling on her fears of Dave leaving her."[11]

Hoping to find a way to reverse this cycle, the therapist conjectured that if Alicia were to stop pursuing Dave, he might become more interested in her. Conversely, if Dave were to show greater interest in Alicia, she might focus less on pursuing him. However, since the therapist observed that "Dave didn't consider himself capable of making changes, given his loss of feelings," he concluded that the couple had only one viable option—to ask Alicia if she would be willing to change her behavior to make Dave more sexually responsive. Would she be willing to reverse course and stop pursuing Dave? As might be expected from the story of Nancy Holt and other women who made sacrifices to save their marriages, Alicia said she would try. Thus, the therapist "suggested that she could forget to kiss him or kiss him and forget to say that she loved him. She might also dress for bed in a way that downplayed her interest in sex. When Dave came home late, she might be so absorbed in some activity that Dave would have to seek *her* attention."[12]

The therapist's next sentence is most revealing. "Because the renewal of Dave's interest in her couldn't be forced, his free will would need to be given time to express itself by Alicia's getting more involved in her own life, going back to work or, as she was an avid reader, joining a book club."[13] What's revealing here is the therapist's sensitivity to the man's possibly threatened "free will," a sensitivity that, according to my sampling of sex therapy's recommended approaches to the incompatibility of heterosexual partners, does not similarly inform the profession's handling of women's disinclination to copulate with men. In studies describing the treatment of heterosexual women's "vaginismus," "frigidity," "inhibited sexual desire," "aversive sexual desire," and "hypoactive sexual desire," therapists typically show less concern for violating women's autonomy. They are more likely to recommend that their women patients recognize and respect masculine "free will" than they are to seek a comparable accommodation of men. Accordingly, in the search for the solution to the problem of Dave and Alicia's mismatched sexual desire, Alicia was the one advised to adjust her behavior—she was asked to modify her performance of sexual interest and availability to better suit Dave's needs.

Sensitivity to a man's free-will is treated as a responsibility of men's wives who, generally speaking, appear in case studies as unlikely to take a confrontational or aggressive stand when they are sexually dissatisfied by their male partners. For example, in a case vignette from a paper on "Male Hypoactive Desire Disorder" (Hall, 2015), published in *Systemic Sex Therapy*, an unhappy wife's effort to rouse her sexually disinterested husband reveals a level of sensitivity and reticence that has no counterpart in case studies when the genders are reversed—when the man is sexually frustrated: "When Marie would timidly raise the subject of sex, [Paul] would initiate, but then Marie would refuse thinking Paul was only initiating because of her complaint and not because he desired her sexually."[14]

In a similar display of sensitivity to a man's needs, when Dave and Alicia's therapist asked Alicia to stop pursuing Dave in the hope of reinvigorating Dave's sexual interest in her, Alicia complied. That strategy seemed to work, at least in the short run, since Dave's sexual feelings for her did return for a while. But the therapist, again showing disproportionate sensitivity to a man, gave equal credit to both partners for this positive outcome, noting that "in essence, they had gotten out of each other's way, allowing themselves to rediscover each other."[15] The truth of the matter is that when Dave had been asked if he would be willing to make changes for Alicia, he declined: "He didn't consider himself capable of making changes." Only one of the partners had agreed to make changes—the woman.

Nadia–Ivan

Like the Dave–Alicia case, the case of Nadia–Ivan concerns a spouse's dissatisfaction with the other's low sexual desire. Most significant, however, these cases resemble each other in sharing the same authors; they also appear next to one another in the same article, "A Catalytic Approach to Brief Therapy" (Fraser and Solovey, 2004). The main difference between these cases is that the genders are reversed. In Dave–Alicia, the man experiences low sexual interest, while in Nadia–Ivan, it's the woman. This singular difference, with everything else held relatively constant, offers a kind of natural experiment addressing questions of how treatment of low sexual interest in a man compares to treatment of low sexual interest in a woman, and how sexual "free will" is conceptualized for men and for women.

In the case of Nadia and Ivan, the couple had been married for almost thirteen years and had two young children, aged four and five. The therapist reports that Nadia said she "felt numb when they made love. Throughout their marriage she had tried to meet Ivan's needs; however, lately he was becoming increasingly frustrated with her over lack of desire. Complaining that they did not have sex frequently enough, Ivan didn't like it when Nadia would just lay there."[16] In explaining why she had not been able to give Ivan the kind of sex he wanted, Nadia reported that "given her responsibilities with the children, she had been more tired lately, and, consequently, she was having more difficulty forcing herself to have sex with her husband."[17] The latter portion of this admission is worth dwelling on. We usually think of sexual coercion as person A forcing person B to receive or perform some unwanted sexual act. With regard to physical force, if person A overpowers B, sexual coercion had obviously occurred. But in the Nadia–Ivan case, the woman claimed she had been "forcing herself to have sex with her husband." What does sexual coercion mean when person B forces herself to receive or perform an unwanted sexual act because she believes she must—because she believes that if she does not comply with person A's request/demand, he will do something unacceptable or even unbearable to her, such as divorce her and take her children? That in turn raises the question whether self-coercion is any less coercive and any less deserving of condemnation than other means of controlling and limiting the victim's sexual choices. The question is important because the most common kind of coercion is the ordinary and nonviolent kind in which a man, often a husband, threatens a woman with a severe, albeit nonviolent, penalty if she refuses to "be natural" and "play the part."[18]

Consider that several weeks before beginning therapy, Nadia and Ivan "had an argument about sex, during which Ivan threatened Nadia with divorce if she didn't get 'her' problem solved."[19] Consider too that the authors observed that "this was especially upsetting for Nadia because Ivan had never threatened to leave her before. Ivan always went by his word, so Nadia knew that if she didn't do something, he was likely to leave."[20] What might have made Ivan's threat even more frightening to Nadia is the fact that she had primary caregiving responsibility for two small boys who were already exhausting her.

This is where gender inequality becomes a problem for sex therapy in its tendency to overlook the matter of a woman's "free will." In the Nadia–Ivan case, as presented in the document, the therapist didn't ask how Ivan's threat to leave might have affected Nadia's feelings for him, her capacity to enjoy sex with him, or her willingness to engage in sex therapy. The case study does not take up the question of whether, under the shadow of Ivan's threat, the notion of Nadia's sexual "consent" makes any sense. The therapist focused instead on Nadia's remote sexual history, specifically, her sexual assault by an adult male living with her family when she was between the ages of thirteen and sixteen. As in the case from the previous chapter of the woman who had been sexually abused as a child by her stepfather, the earlier trauma received therapeutic attention as the one and only source of the wife's alleged sexual dysfunction. As the therapist explained to Ivan:

the problem that Nadia is experiencing is not only about your ability as a lover. As you know, Nadia was abused as a young girl. As part of that abuse she became turned off to sex. This is not at all uncommon for women who have been abused, and in fact Nadia's reaction was quite expected. This business of being turned off has to do with mental associations that Nadia has about sex. . . . Pleasurable fantasies within a trusting relationship with you are what Nadia needs to feel turned on.[21]

Nadia had been adamant about her need to save her marriage, and she had been quite clear about her disinterest in sex. But the therapist appeared to hear something different. He concluded that Nadia's primary need now, as an adult, was "to discover the power of sexual pleasure in a trusting and loving marriage."[22] The therapist "then proceeded to unfold a plan for therapy that included many elements of Masters and Johnson's work. He explained to Ivan that the course of treatment would involve a sacrifice from him . . . an initial prohibition against intercourse while they engaged in a program of progressive pleasuring,"[23] a program that should slowly advance from talking without touching, to touching while clothed, and then to touching without clothes, each step becoming more sexually intimate until, finally, the therapist instructed Nadia to engage in intercourse: "to insert Ivan's erect penis into her vagina so she can feel the power of eventually reducing it to a withering pulp."[24] Nadia had not expressed an interest in gaining pleasure from intercourse, nor had she expressed an interest in reducing a man's penis "to a withering pulp." According to the case record, the therapist simply assumed that this was what she wanted and needed.

On follow-up, a month later, Nadia reported that she "was experiencing pleasure with sex (both on her own and with Ivan), and Ivan was no longer contemplating divorce."[25] The therapist took this as an indicator that Nadia's sexual disinterest/aversion had been resolved, and his interpretation may have been entirely correct. Perhaps Nadia did need to discuss the details of the sexual trauma she had experienced as an adolescent; perhaps she needed to put it behind her. She might have also needed the program of Masters and Johnson sexual exercises to help her discover her latent capacity for sexual pleasure.

Alternatively, it is possible that Nadia was faking—faking sexual pleasure with Ivan—much as Nancy Holt faked the belief that her marriage was egalitarian. Perhaps marriage for Nadia had become a place where, as Adrienne Rich put it, a woman "learned to adapt to male domination out of necessity," and that "sexual adaptation—learning to 'be natural and play the part'"—was simply the price she paid for survival.[26]

Once again, we will never know for sure why Nadia expressed sexual pleasure, whether her claims were genuine or not. All we know is that in this case study, the authors do not direct readers' attention to the possibility that Nadia's long-standing sexual pattern ("Nadia didn't like sex . . . [but] throughout their marriage she had tried to meet Ivan's needs"[27]) was replicated and reinforced in and by sex therapy. The authors did not document the *possibility* that Nadia was only going through the motions to preserve her marriage and to make her husband and therapist happy. Finally, the authors of the Dave–Alicia and Nadia–Ivan case studies did not note that they handled the issue of low sexual desire differently when it was a woman who presented with low sexual interest. In both instances, the man was given a pass, regardless of his high or low sexual interest, and in both, the woman was asked to change; she was asked to accommodate her husband's needs.

Double-Consciousness

One way to explain these gender differences is through empirical studies that show that those who have greater power are generally less adaptable. They have more difficulty taking the other's perspective.[28] While those with less power—those who belong to subordinated groups, such as blacks and women—are more adaptable. As underdogs, they must learn to take others' perspective; their very survival may depend on it. W. E. B. Du Bois called this ability, "double-consciousness," and described it as the "sense of always looking at one's self through the eyes of others."[29] "Double-consciousness" may explain why women are considered more adaptable to men's behavior and feelings than men are to women's behavior and feelings, and why therapists appear to assume that because women are (or should be) better at understanding and adapting to men than vice versa, they should take the lead in accommodating.

To provide an example of this gender bias, consider "Relationship Enhancement Therapy: A Case Study for Treatment of Vaginismus: Therapy," (Harmon, Waldo, and Johnson, 1994), an article published in the peer-reviewed *Family Journal: Counseling and Therapy for Couples and Families*. That study purports to show sex therapy professionals how to help a young couple with a sexual problem—in this case, the wife's "vaginismus"—improve their communication skills. The specific helping technique demonstrated in the article involves coaching the partners to "express emotions, thoughts and desires clearly and honestly without generating unnecessary hostility and defensiveness."[30] What readers should note, however, is the article's one-sided focus on helping the wife empathize with her husband—how it provides a detailed example of how to coach her to empathize with her husband's hurt feelings after she refuses sex with him, but provides no complementary demonstration of how to coach her husband to empathize with her. Indeed, from my survey of the sex therapy literature, I could not find any studies focused on helping heterosexual males empathize with female partners who find sex aversive and/or refuse their partner's sexual advances.

The therapy session involves a newly married couple, Dawn and Tim, both aged twenty-one, who began sex therapy because of dissatisfaction with their sex life.[31] Dawn is a woman who experiences low levels of sexual desire but seemingly only feels distressed about it when her husband complains. Contrary to what the authors of the *DSM* seem to indicate, Dawn is not unusual in reporting that she is satisfied with little or no sexual activity. Research tells us that low sexual desire is not generally troubling for women, except, that is, when a woman with low sexual desire has a male partner whose desires are incompatible with hers. Then her equanimity disappears.[32] The association between her low sexual desire and distress often spikes, becoming significant and substantial as it increases to more than four times the level of distress experienced by single women with low desire. The transcript of this session provides an opportunity to inquire into why women with low sexual desire tend to feel higher levels of distress when partnered with men,[33] as well as an opportunity to examine how sex therapy pressures women to adapt to men's sexual needs—how, for sex therapy, it may not be as simple as "no means no" when a wife attempts to reject her husband's sexual overtures. She must also try to understand his hurt feelings.

TIM [*to Dawn*]: I sometimes get disturbed when you don't want to have sex, and I guess sometimes that you're rejecting me. I sometimes feel that you do it a lot.

DAWN: You're disturbed when I don't want to have sex and you feel like I'm rejecting you. Is that as a person or as a sexual person?

MALE THERAPIST [*to Dawn*]: Just show understanding to what he is saying.

DAWN: Well, I'm unclear on what he's saying. I don't understand.

MALE THERAPIST: You've got what he's said so far; that was beautiful. Now if you would just stop and [*to Tim*] you could go on.

TIM: That's how I feel sometimes. Sometimes I feel real confused. I think—why don't you want to have sex, why don't you want to have sex more often? Sometimes I don't understand why I get excited a lot and you don't get as excited as I.

MALE THERAPIST [TO TIM]: That's great. Could you add any emotion that causes in you?

TIM: I'm not sure I know. I think confusion. Is that an emotion?

MALE THERAPIST: Could there be hurt?

TIM: Uh . . . no not always. Well, yeah, sometimes.

DAWN: Well what does the word rejection mean?

MALE THERAPIST: Dawn, this isn't the time to question.

DAWN: Well, you're asking him about feelings. When he said rejection, you said hurt, and he said no. So what does he feel when he feels rejected—just nothing?

TIM: Well, it's not that I'm rejected right now. It's just that sometimes I'm really confused when you don't want to have sex as often as I do, why you're not as sexual as me.

DAWN: So you don't understand why I don't want to have sex as much as you? (Dawn's tone strongly suggested impatience).

FEMALE THERAPIST [TO DAWN]: On the cue card here, it says understanding and patience.

DAWN: I don't understand.

FEMALE THERAPIST: You're not able to do that?

DAWN: No, I don't understand. I keep looking at that [the cue card] and I don't understand how he feels, I guess.

FEMALE THERAPIST: You mean when he tells you he feels hurt, you don't understand?

DAWN: Right, in the sexual sense. How can I understand that?[34]

From the transcript, the therapists appear to be advising Dawn on Tim's needs, asking her to show more understanding and acceptance of his hurt and confusion following her refusal to have sex with him. At the end of the quoted passage, when Dawn asks Tim about how well he understands *her* feelings ("So you don't understand why I don't want to have sex as much as you?"), the therapist immediately redirected her back to Tim's feelings ("On the cue card here, it says understanding and patience"). Indeed, whenever Dawn interrupted the focus on Tim's needs, whenever she tried to ask questions or assert her own priorities, the therapists redirected her back to Tim, telling her to "just show understanding of what he is saying," or "Dawn, this isn't the time to question," or simply, "Now if you would just stop."

Masculine Exceptionalism

As a final example of how differently a man may be treated in the professional literature, consider the case of Ron, aged twenty-six, and Deb, aged twenty-two, described in the article, "Sexless Marriages and Sex Therapy" (Renshaw, 1995), which appeared in *Case Studies in Sex Therapy*. Like Nick and Susan, Ron and Deb began sex therapy because Deb threatened to leave if Ron did not become more sexually responsive. This threat must have seemed very real to Ron since Deb had left him once before for a couple of months for the same reasons. At that time, after Deb returned to Ron, he did appear more sexually responsive for a while, but only for a while. As Deb described the current status of their sexual relationship during sex therapy, "for the last year it's back to zero sex."[35] Ron claimed that his sexual reticence resulted from a trauma that occurred a year before their marriage. His then girlfriend, Joan, with whom he was deeply in love and who was carrying his child, died in an accidental house fire. Although Deb consoled Ron in his grief and fell in love with him, Ron claimed he wasn't over Joan's death. In a joint session with Deb, Ron confessed his continuing preoccupation with his loss, to which Deb responded in sobs, "How can I compete with someone who is dead? I've always worried that he looks at me and wishes I was her."[36]

Ron and Deb opted to continue seeing their therapist, and, as before, their sex life seemed to improve for a while: "In the next 3 weeks the couple reported having 'the best sex ever' in their relationship."[37] But that changed quickly when Deb began talking of having a baby. "Ron's face whitened, his eyes glazed, he became withdrawn and could not discuss it."[38] The therapist offered to see Ron individually, but he declined and dropped out of treatment. As the therapist explained,

> his griefwork was obviously incomplete, but he was not ready to continue. This decision must be respected. There are limitations to the pace and directions of therapeutic change. Each individual is different. The therapist can only stand by and offer an open door.[39]

The common factor in the Susan–Nick and Ron–Deb cases is the wife pressuring the husband to begin therapy. In both cases, the frustrated wife threatens to leave if her husband does not become more sexually responsive and accommodating. What these cases also have in common is that the wife's threat proves toothless. The husband withdraws from therapy and the therapist's involvement in the case ends in "respect" for this masculine exercise of "free will," perhaps illustrating how much easier it is for a husband than a wife to remain unaffected by the "low sexual desire" label. Because of this professional respect, when a husband is diagnosed with low sexual desire, he seems more likely to back out of treatment, in effect telling his wife and therapist, "Take it or leave it, this is who I am." As one therapist noted in "Hidden Disorder/Hidden Desire: Presentations of Low Sexual Desire in Men" (2014), an article from the fifth edition of *Principles and Practice of Sex Therapy*, after an unsuccessful attempt at treating a husband's sexual indifference to his wife, "the case of Brad and Stacey reminds therapists that some problems of desire may not be amenable to intervention."[40] Slowly and painfully, Stacy and the therapist came to realize that Brad's sexual desire could not be rekindled, Brad dropped out of treatment, and the partners decided to separate.

Sex therapists readily acknowledge many times and occasions when an individual cannot be trained, stimulated, or guided into feeling sexual attraction for another. As Frost and Donovan (2015) explained, "sexual desire has been considered notoriously difficult to treat by clinicians from many backgrounds, including psychology, psychiatry, and gynecology."[41] However, as a field, sex therapy has yet to examine how the gender divide makes some cases of impaired sexual desire more difficult to solve than others. Sexual desire problems among heterosexual men, while less common than those among heterosexual women, are also less amenable to treatment. In general, heterosexual men experiencing low desire are less open to making adjustments to suit a heterosexual partner's sexual needs. This observation, drawn from this survey of case studies, is confirmed by a recent study of thirty-one heterosexual couples in long-term marriages (Elliot and Umberson, 2008). While the wives interviewed for this study said they would try to increase their interest in sex and the frequency of sexual activity to please their spouse, comparatively few men exhibited the same flexibility. As the study's authors reported,

> husbands who are less sexual than their wives described increasing difficulty getting and maintaining an erection with age and view this as a physiological problem. As Harold (African American, age 61, married 32 years) puts it, "the plumbing doesn't work." On the face of it, Viagra would seem to provide an effective pharmaceutical substitute for performing desire. Yet, in general, they are reluctant to take this step, in part because of the embarrassment of seeing a doctor, but also, in large part, as Jim's comments reveal, because of a genuine lack of sexual interest.[42]

Heterosexual men, according to the evidence of case studies, not only present as more sexually intransigent than heterosexual women, their sexual intransigence appears more readily accepted by spouses and therapists as "genuine." Men reporting low sexual desire appear less inclined to follow their therapist's treatment program and less inclined to make the kinds of changes their partner seeks. In general, a man's position in his marital orbit does not readily adapt to his wife's sexual or emotional needs. Her position adapts to his.[43]

8
Women's Duty

I think about sex all the time, not because I have a high sex drive but because it hurts when I have intercourse. As soon as my husband comes home from work, I worry because I'm afraid he'll ask me to make love and I won't want to because of the pain. It isn't that I don't love him. I do. I feel guilty because I am constantly looking for excuses not to have sex with him but I can't help it because it hurts so much. He tries to understand but it's been over a year now and his patience has worn thin.
—Jo Marie Kessler, "When the Diagnosis is Vaginismus" (1988)

I can continue . . . with sexual intercourse although I'm in pain . . . I do . . . because I think it will somehow . . . he thinks it's nice . . . and, like, he will come soon . . . and I . . . I like . . . I continue because he will come soon . . . because it feels like . . . it is really foolish to feel like that . . . but you do . . . you don't want to interrupt it . . . for his sake.
—Interview with anonymous subject, Elmerstig et al., "Why Do Young Women Continue to Have Sexual Intercourse Despite Pain?" (2008)

Reproduction has historically been one of the main purposes of marriage. Intercourse in marriage, therefore, given its connection to reproduction, has long been regarded as obligatory, and a wife's failure to live up to this obligation, whether for reasons of discomfort or pain, or any other reason, has often been treated as grounds for divorce or annulment. As recently as 1973, in an article titled, "Wives Who Refuse Their Husbands," a physician cautioned that a wife's "refusal to have intercourse is often the first step in a . . . campaign to drive toward divorce." In line with this, one of the most common reasons women give for trying to resolve their inability to perform intercourse has been their wish to have children. For example, in the case study, "Sex Is a Nasty Business," which originally appeared in the *DSM-III-R Case Book* (1989), and then was reproduced in the *DSM-IV Case Book* (1994), and the *DSM-IV-TR Case Book* (2002), a wife, Clara, was said to have an intense dislike of sex in all its forms, and a particular aversion to intercourse ("She never looks forward to sexual contact with her husband and actively discourages his advances"). At the same time, she wanted to correct "her problem" because "her husband has been pressuring her to become pregnant again. She would like to become pregnant both to please him and because she herself wants another child."[1] To say this another way, Clara and her husband both wanted to overcome Clara's aversion to sex to solve their family/relational problem.

This is what I wish to highlight now: how women's resistance to sex with men is often seen, in sex therapy's professional literature, as an obstacle to achieving family goals, and how overcoming that resistance—taking on the burden of unwanted intercourse—is treated as a responsible way of "saving the marriage" and "protecting the family."

She Takes One for the Team

Mary, as she was described in "Treating Women's Orgasmic Difficulties" (Carpenter et al., 2017), published in *The Wiley Handbook of Sex Therapy* (according to a Wiley advertisement, "a comprehensive and empirically-based review of the latest theory and practice in the psychotherapeutic treatment of sexual problems"[2]), had been married for about thirty-nine years when she was diagnosed with ovarian cancer. Her treatment included a total hysterectomy, the removal of her ovaries and fallopian tubes, and eight cycles of chemotherapy. Prior to treatment, Mary and her husband had engaged in intercourse and other sexual activities two to four times per week throughout their marriage. However, after Mary's genital and reproductive system trauma, she said she could no longer enjoy intercourse. The problem this created for her, she explained, is that "her relationship with her partner was beginning to suffer." She said she "'shut down' during sexual activity, and said she would become distressed to the point of 'sobbing' during and following sexual encounters. She stated that her husband was kind, gentle, and supportive but was 'at a loss' and ready to 'shut the door on [their] sex life.'"[3]

Mary's treatment, according to the case report, had a single aim: to restore her capacity to enjoy intercourse. Thus, sessions one and two involved muscle relaxation training "to help reduce overall anxiety and improve control over muscles of the pelvic floor and throughout the body. Recommendations were made for improving vaginal health (e.g., use of vaginal moisturizers, Kegel exercises) with instructions for ongoing home practice."[4] Sessions three to six were devoted to a series of "self-exploration/mindfulness exercises aimed at increasing awareness of pleasant bodily sensations."[5] Sessions seven to nine "focused on identifying conditions that made sexual activity more satisfying," and sessions ten to twelve "focused on goal-setting and relapse prevention."[6]

The treatment outcome: Mary said she could once again experience orgasm through intercourse and rated her overall sex life as "above average." While she claimed she continued to have "maladaptive cognitions" during sexual activity, they appeared less frequently, and she reported she was "better able to identify them as inaccurate, exaggerated, or unhelpful, and to generate alternatives."[7]

I placed this case under the subheading, "She Takes One for the Team" because Mary's main motivation for initiating sex therapy treatment following cancer treatments, as described in the case study, did not include any wish to restore her pleasure in intercourse. This sixty-three-year-old post-operative cancer patient didn't need intercourse for herself. Rather, her concern was for her husband—how her inability to perform intercourse was hurting her relationship with him. She said she "missed the closeness she enjoyed following sexual activity throughout their marriage and was feeling hopeless that she would ever experience it again."[8] But the question of Mary's "closeness" to her husband was not included in the treatment plan. There is no record of the therapist addressing the issue of "closeness." Only Mary's sexual responses were addressed, which may explain why her husband didn't participate in treatment. The relationship problem that brought this cancer patient to sex therapy was reconceptualized as her sexual problem, a matter of her individual psychopathy, thus her diagnosis, "female orgasmic disorder."

A similar kind of overlooking of the relational disorder is apparent in the treatment of Alice, aged thirty-six, the mother of two young daughters. Alice's case appeared in the article, "Inhibited Arousal in Women" (Wylie, 2015), published in *Systemic Sex Therapy*, a volume intended for "the many clinicians who want to progress to a more comprehensive and integrative understanding of sexual dysfunctions."[9] Alice had no interest in sex with her husband. She told her therapist she "would be quite happy to never engage in sex [with her husband] again." Why then did she begin sex therapy? It was to "correct the poor couple image that her daughters were receiving from them. 'They never see us being warm,' she commented. 'They don't know how parents should be. They are getting old enough to comment on couple behavior on TV and compare it to their experience at home.'"[10] While the therapist's expressed goal was to help Alice overcome her disinterest in sex, Alice's goal was to nurture her daughters' relational skills; she wanted to provide a more positive role model for them. As in Mary's case, the relationship problem that brought Alice to therapy was reconceptualized as Alice's sexual problem, thus her diagnosis, "female sexual interest/arousal disorder."

"Treating Genital Pain Associated with Sexual Intercourse" (Meana et al., 2017) published in the *Wiley Handbook of Sex Therapy*, similarly diagnoses a couple's relationship problem as a woman's individual need for sexual treatment. Like Mary, Kari found intercourse unpleasant and even painful, and her inability to enjoy intercourse made her husband, Greg, very unhappy, for it "confirmed Greg's suspicion that Kari was simply not attracted to him and that she did not really want to have sex with him."[11] As in Mary's case, the only treatment alternative offered was helping Kari become more accepting of and responsive to intercourse. As the case is presented in the *Handbook*, the husband's insecurity about his sexual attractiveness does not become a topic of discussion or a target of treatment. The therapist doesn't ask the husband if he can manage without intercourse, or if there are other ways he might be reassured about his self-worth, or if he would be willing to make accommodations of any kind. Instead, when Greg was consulted, it was to help determine which kinds of therapeutic interventions should be performed on his wife. When the sex therapist talked with Greg, it was about how to manage what were presumed to be Kari's problems: they "discussed treatment options . . . ranging from the minimally invasive application of lidocaine to the maximally invasive surgery, with a recommendation of cognitive-behavioral therapy (CBT)/pain management regardless of the somatic treatment chosen."[12]

Among the most striking differences between Mary's case and that of Kari–Greg is that Kari, Greg, and the therapist assume that, no matter what treatment option was selected for Kari, intercourse would remain uncomfortable. Accordingly, they did not discuss how to make Kari's intercourse experience pleasurable or orgasmic. A second difference is Greg's motivation for intercourse; it seemed centered in his insecurities, grounded in his belief that being denied access to penetrative sex signals that Kari was "not attracted to him." Finally, since none of the verbal and noninvasive interventions succeeded in making intercourse more tolerable for Kari, she agreed to go ahead with major vaginal surgery—a vestibulectomy—which involved the removal of her hymen, mucous membrane, and Bartholin glands ducts. Unfortunately, that was unsuccessful too. Even after surgery, Kari continued to experience pain: "The couple's hopes that intercourse would be completely painless were not fulfilled, but they felt satisfied that they had tried everything available."[13]

Finally, a 1989 article, "The Treatment of Vaginismus" (Leiblum et al., 1989), published in *Principles and Practice of Sex Therapy*, describes a wife who began therapy "at the insistence of her husband, who threatened to leave unless she got some help with her problem."[14] "Her problem," according to her husband, is that she did not enjoy sex and refused intercourse. From her side, although she wanted to become a more satisfying sex partner for her husband so he would not leave her, she "resented his labeling her as the problem, and believed that his lack of warmth contributed to it."[15]

The authors did not describe the therapy as an effort to *train* the wife to become a more agreeable sex partner for her husband, but neither did they report any efforts to make sex pleasurable for her, and no mention was made of efforts directed to changing the husband, who was reportedly only minimally involved in treatment; for example, he refused to participate in sensate focus exercises, explaining that to do so "would be giving her what she wanted—physical closeness but not sex."[16] No one decided that his refusal to do something to please his wife is a relationship problem. By default, then, the wife was the avenue selected for solving the relationship problem.

The early sessions focused on helping her get used to inserting "penile-shaped objects" into her vagina. During later sessions, she was introduced to the therapy technique associated with Wolpe and Lazarus: systematic desensitization. This involved asking her to imagine inserting her finger into her vagina, followed by a tampon, and then her husband's penis while she attempted to relax.[17] In the fantasy phase of these exercises, to reduce her fear that her husband's large penis would tear her relatively small vagina, "she was asked to imagine herself as possessing an almost cavernous vagina which could incorporate a penis without difficulty whatsoever."[18] Finally, the therapist had the wife insert dilators into her vagina to increase its width and desensitize her to penetration.

The therapist asked the wife to refrain from attempting intercourse at home until she became more comfortable with the idea, but her husband insisted, and after four weeks of persistent effort, "he was able to achieve partial penetration."[19] This pleased him, and although he felt she was beginning to make progress—her fear and revulsion were not nearly as intense—she "continued to want him to ejaculate quickly and also continued to fear that his large penis could not fit entirely into her vagina."[20] While the husband claimed he succeeded in getting almost the full length of his penis into his wife's vagina prior to the final therapy session, the authors of the study judged the wife's success merely "erratic," since she said she could only tolerate her husband inserting his penis halfway into her vagina, and only when he was at the point of ejaculation, "to get it over with."[21]

Ten weeks later, a follow-up session revealed that the couple's intercourse frequency had increased to two or three times weekly, "occasionally with full penetration and at times with approximately two-thirds penetration."[22] The wife said this outcome was fine with her, but the husband wasn't happy. He said he wanted intercourse more often, and wanted oral sex too, which she was unwilling to perform. As for the study's authors, they viewed the case as a "partial success." The couple was now having intercourse on a routine basis. That was the positive part. But on the negative side, "they continued to have difficulties with full penetration and . . . continued [to have] difficulties in working out a mutually satisfactory sexual and marital relationship."[23]

This case study calls attention to the ways in which "sex therapy" normalizes heterosexual women's willingness to make sacrifices for the benefit of the husband. It also calls attention to how sex therapy may closely resemble training women to function as a husband's sex object. Such an equation is naturalized by the belief that a wife should be able to accept her spouse's penis into her vagina. If she can't do it, the therapeutic logic follows, she can be taught to do it.

Who Owns Mrs. D.'s Vagina?

It is often very difficult to identify the ultimate rationale for encouraging a woman to engage in painful, unrewarding intercourse beyond the therapist's and couple's belief that it is the wife's duty and the husband's right. Andrea Dworkin explains:

> Penetration is taken to be a use, not an abuse: a normal use; it is appropriate to enter her. . . . She is human, of course, but by the standard that does not include physical privacy, since to keep a man out altogether and for a lifetime is deviant in the extreme, a psychopathology, a repudiation of the way she is expected to manifest her humanity.[24]

In the case of Mrs. D., the cultural belief that a woman's vagina should be receptive to her spouse's penis is treated as a self-evident truth, requiring little or no justification. This is the dominant storyline of an article about Mrs. D., aged forty-one, and her husband, Mr. D., aged fifty-two, that appeared in the *Journal of Sex & Marital Therapy* titled, "Marriage Consummated after 22 Years: A Case Report" (Chakrabarti and Sinha, 2002). According to the article, Mrs. D. was highly distressed and guilt-ridden over having "deprived" her husband of his "conjugal rights" for more than twenty years. She offered to give him a divorce so he could marry a normal woman, but Mr. D. declined. He was described as a "normal and supportive husband who said that remarriage was out of the question. He felt that the problem was theirs to resolve as a couple."[25]

Mrs. D.'s treatment began with a prescription of sertraline (an anti-anxiety medication), followed by four sessions with a psychiatrist, each session separated by a two-day interval. The first session was largely devoted to "explaining normal human reproductive anatomy and physiology, including the stages of intercourse," and ended with the psychiatrist advising the couple "to indulge in foreplay over the next 2 days without penetration." During the second session, the couple was advised to go home and "practice mutual masturbation with finger penetration, over the next 2 days." And during the third session, the couple was advised to go home and "attempt to consummate their marriage over the next 2 days."[26]

During the fourth and final session, "the couple reported consummation of the marriage with full penile penetration of the vagina and ejaculation within the vagina." The wife claimed that intercourse was not so very bad after all, since she "found the pain insignificant compared to what she had previously imagined it to be."[27]

What Mrs. D.'s treatment illustrates is how, according to current sex therapy practice, a wife's vagina continues to be treated as shared property, owned by both the husband and wife. As Jeanne Shaw (1994) remarked in her article, "Treatment of Primary Vaginismus: A New Perspective," a nonresistant, compliant woman, thus takes the stance, "My vagina belongs to you, too. I relinquish sole ownership in order to feel like a normal woman to have normal sex for my normal partner."[28]

Mrs. D. believed she owed access to her vagina to her husband, her husband believed she owed access to her vagina to him, and the therapist and authors of the study, to all appearances, believed it too—all without signs of ill will. Indeed, everyone seemed very respectful and sympathetic to Mrs. D. during every phase of treatment, which perhaps shows that even the most misogynistic and pernicious gender ideologies can be sustained by thought and action that do not appear misogynist or pernicious to the participants or other observers. A husband who appears to be caring and ethical, such as Mr. D., as well as caring and ethical therapists, can hold women to false and spurious sexual obligations, too.

Denying the Possibility of Sexual Coercion

Even in these enlightened "post-feminist" times, sex therapists may accept as normal and natural heterosexual women's obligation to adapt to men's sexual needs, while disavowing heterosexual men's complementary obligation to adapt to women's sexual or relational needs. A husband can be excused from the responsibility of meeting his wife's sexual/relational needs if that responsibility makes him feel uncomfortable or coerced. By contrast, as represented by the record of case studies, therapists often appear unattuned to the possibility that their female patients are experiencing coercion. In particular, they tend to ignore the role that men's and women's socio-economic inequality plays in their sexual interactions, and sometimes go so far as to overtly support that inequality by denying a woman a voice in her own therapy sessions, even when she explicitly complains of feeling pressured to engage in sex she really does not want.

The next case study originally appeared in an article titled, "Sexual Aversion Disorder" (Janata and Kingsberg, 2005), published in the *Handbook of Sexual Dysfunction*, a text that purportedly "provides the clinician reader with a practical, commonsense guide to treatment planning that treats the patient as an individual rather than as a disease entity."[29] I include it here because, like many other case studies, it illustrates how sex therapy, in its preoccupation with facilitating women's copulation with men, overlooks the possibility of sexual coercion.

I also include it here because, like other case studies, it provides almost no information on the woman's motivation to enter into sex therapy, including whether it was her voluntary choice to begin or a "choice" forced upon her.[30] What we do learn, however, is that Joyce, much like Nadia from the previous chapter, had a history of sexual victimization that went back to her childhood. A seventeen-year-old male neighbor had raped her when she was twelve. As the therapist reports, "the abuse continued for about 2 years until, at age 14, she threatened to inform his parents of his actions and he ceased his abuse of her."[31] We also learn that Joyce met her future husband, Bill, at the age of twenty-eight, was initially attracted to him, and experienced arousal and orgasm when they first had intercourse. At some point, however, a point not specified in the case study, sex with him became distinctly unpleasant. The authors go on to say that Joyce "decided to 'tough it out,' assuming, she supposed in retrospect, that her sexual response would improve given enough time and love."[32] But it did not improve. "On the contrary, Bill became increasingly frustrated with her avoidance of sex and demanded more frequent intercourse."[33] Joyce attempted to explain her aversion to her husband's sexual overtures, but he did not respond with understanding and compassion. To the contrary, he "became irritated and verbally abusive."[34]

The therapist addressed the husband's irritation and verbal abuse only indirectly. Instead of discussing these issues with Bill (and Joyce), as problems in need of a solution, the therapist tried to temper Bill's angry reactions by appealing to his compassion. The therapist asked Joyce to tell her husband how she had been raped as a child as an explanation for her sexual reluctance. According to the case study, "this revelation evoked some sensitivity to Joyce's [sexual] response from Bill and temporarily tempered his insistence on intercourse,"[35] but apparently the revelation had no lasting effect. His insistence on intercourse returned, in the same intemperate fashion, a phenomenon that was still not directly addressed by the therapist. How was the husband insisting? Was he forcing penetration? Was he raping her? The case study does not suggest that these possibilities were explored in therapy. Instead, Joyce was placed on a program of systematic desensitization, the kind of program associated with Joseph Wolpe, Charles Lazarus, and other behaviorists, whereby a patient is given a hierarchy of fear-provoking sexual scenarios, ranging from masturbation to intercourse, and asked to relax while she imagines each one in the hope of extinguishing the association between those scenarios and fear. The case study ends rather vaguely with a reference to the couple's resumption of "healthier" sexual interactions: "Fifteen sessions conducted over a period of 5 months were needed to help Joyce and Bill resume the healthier sexual life that had characterized their early history."[36]

The central questions raised by this case are similar to the ones raised by the Mary, Kari–Gregg, Nadia–Ivan cases and, indeed, to almost all the others raised in this book: Why was little attention paid to the ways Bill interacted with Joyce?

Why wasn't more attention paid to the social/relational context of the couple's marriage? Why didn't the therapist ask Joyce how Bill's verbal abuse and insistence on intercourse might have affected her sexual desire? One of the most discomforting answers that the therapist might have discovered, if those questions had been asked, is that Joyce's sexual aversion was a reaction to Bill's mistreatment of her, a hypothesis well worth exploring, given the fact that Joyce claimed her aversion to sex began during her marriage to Bill and that Bill's history of emotional abuse during sexual activity emerged during therapy sessions. The possibility that he had been mistreating Joyce, possibly raping her, may, like Ivan's threats to Nadia, have been dismissed by the therapist because Bill was the therapist's "ally" in the sense of restoring sexual "health" to the relationship. He had the same goal for Joyce that the therapist had: to make her more sexually active and responsive. Like the Nadia–Ivan case, a therapist's preoccupation with reigniting a woman's sexual life with her husband may have overwhelmed all other considerations, most critically the question of the woman's personal autonomy and integrity.

Denying the Reality of Sexual Coercion

As noted in an earlier chapter, sex therapy in the 1960s encouraged a husband to force penetration with the justification that this was the only way to cure his wife's psychiatric disorder, "vaginismus." In the Nadia–Ivan and Joyce–Bill cases, the therapists overlooked the possibility that their female patient might have been forced to play the part of the sexually satisfied, agreeable wife to ensure the survival of her marriage, a finding that is, again, entirely consistent with Elliott and Umberson's study of long-term marriages:

> Many of the wives we interviewed experience themselves as less sexual than their husbands, yet they view sexual frequency as a barometer of a good marriage, as do their husbands.... In addition to housework, childcare, and paid work, employed wives often feel compelled to show affection to their partners by having sex with them.[37]

The following case study, from an article titled, "Treating Inhibited Sexual Desire: A Marital Therapy Approach" (Fish et al., 1984), is similar to the Joyce–Bill case because it too involves coercion.[38] In this case, however, the issue of forced intercourse is no longer hypothetical; it was explicitly acknowledged by the husband, wife, and therapist.

Brad and Lisa, the married couple seeking treatment in this case, had been living together for six years when therapy began. According to the authors, the presenting problem was

Lisa's secondary, situational ISD (Inhibited Sexual Desire) and their constant arguments about sex. Lisa would have been content to never have sex, whereas Brad desired sex at least three times a week. At the beginning of treatment, Lisa and Brad were engaging in sexual intercourse once a month and this was only accomplished through Brad physically forcing Lisa to comply.[39]

But "physically forcing Lisa to comply" was never identified as the problem. Lisa's sexual disinterest in Brad was defined as the problem, and the goal of therapy—the only overt goal according to the published version of the case—was to transform her disinterest into sexual desire: "During the 18 weekly sessions with this couple, Lisa's ISD gradually faded. Initially abhorrent of sex with Brad, Lisa became more tolerant, eventually 'not minding' sex, and finally initiating sex with desire."[40]

The therapist succeeded in getting Lisa to a point where she was "initiating sex with desire" by crafting a bargain with Brad: "during the fifth session, the therapist told Brad that it would be impossible to change Lisa's symptom without his help. He agreed to stop all physical abuse in exchange for the potential of his wife's desire and signed a contract stating so."[41] The therapist treated Brad's violence as counterproductive and self-defeating. When asked to stop expressing his desire with violence, he complied. But Brad's contract to stop sexually assaulting Lisa was defined as a method to "change Lisa's symptom." Brad was not asked to stop forcing Lisa to have sex (the word "rape" was never used) because force is wrong; he was asked to stop forcing Lisa as an act of therapeutic support—because "it would be impossible to change Lisa's symptom without his help" and because it interfered with his realizing his own goal—to have Lisa desire sex with him. Needless to say, Brad got something out of this. He agreed to stop raping Lisa as part of a quid pro quo that involved Lisa agreeing to behave as if she desired him. He traded rape "in exchange for the potential of his wife's desire," and, for a time, it seemed to work. As the authors described the contract's effect, "during the session following Brad's written commitment, Lisa admitted to having sex with Brad after he asked for it, and 'not minding' this sexual contact." By the end of their therapy, they were having sex about twice a week. Brad "learned to ask for what he needed in a way that encouraged Lisa to acquiesce," and "both were satisfied with the frequency of sexual contacts when therapy terminated."[42]

The therapist appeared to assume that Lisa's stream of sexual desire had to get back into its streambed and resume its natural flow. And that may explain why Brad's sexual violence was never taken seriously. It may have been dismissed because Brad's first priority, like the therapist's, was to get Lisa sexually active again. For both, the need to get Lisa to agree to copulate willingly and frequently may have overridden all possible reservations. And this may explain why neither the therapist, the study's authors, nor the editors of the journal that published the article, the *American Journal of Family Therapy*, identified sexual violence as the key to this couple's treatment. Among the many therapists and scholars who have cited this article, not one noted anything sexist or anomalous about it. Rather, it has been interpreted like other sex therapy articles appearing in peer-reviewed journals on the topic of inhibited sexual desire, as an authoritative, objective resource on how to perform therapy for women and couples experiencing inhibited sexual desire. To all intents and purposes, this case, and the way it describes therapy, has represented exemplary practice in the field of sex therapy. Because the authors gloss over the wife's sexual victimization in order to get her to copulate with her spouse, this case may well serve as an exemplar of something else— doublethink, a willingness not only to say that black is white, but also "the ability to *believe* that black is white, and more, to *know* that black is white, and to forget that one has ever believed the contrary."[43]

The therapist in this case might not have overtly affirmed Lisa's obligation to satisfy Brad's sexual needs, but in the service of curing her psychiatric dysfunction—her "inhibited sexual desire"—that is what happened. The central and most unfortunate feature of the therapeutic preoccupation with curing Lisa's alleged psychiatric dysfunction is that it appears to have obscured the harmful effects of Brad's sexual violence. It might also have obscured the possibility that Lisa's unwillingness to have intercourse with her rapist, far from being a sign of a psychiatric disorder, may have been an indicator of Lisa's personal integrity. Her resistance may have been a sign of her mental health.[44]

9
Sex Therapy Without Male Privilege and Power

> If partners can acknowledge differences in sensitive areas, money and status, for example, and discuss the meaning of such differences openly, without trying to redress the imbalance, they will not be as likely to surface in the bedroom disguised as sexual incompatibility.
> —Marny Hall, "Sex Therapy with Lesbian Couples" (1987)

Freud showed no hesitation when it came to dominating Dora. Whenever he and Dora disagreed, Freud smoothly and quickly solved the impasse: he assumed he was right and Dora wrong. When Dora reported being sexually assaulted by Herr K. at the age of thirteen, Freud did not question Herr K.'s behavior; rather, he questioned Dora's rejection of him—her feelings of disgust and anger. Freud showed no interest in analyzing these pro-male biases, and, in fact, it probably didn't occur to him that he might have been biased. This pattern seems to have prevailed with Freud's successors, and, indeed, throughout the history of sex therapy. It's not only that therapists supported men's sexual techniques and preferences over women's; it's that, for the most part, they did not appear to recognize that they were supporting men's interests over women's interests.

A Focus on Inequality

The question this chapter addresses is what sex therapy looks like when men are not involved as patients and partners. As a way of controlling for pro-male bias, this chapter asks how professional wisdom about sex therapy with lesbians might differ from sex therapy recommendations for heterosexuals. The first example is a case study from Marny Hall's "Therapy with Lesbian Couples" (1987) originally published in the peer-reviewed *Journal of Homosexuality*:

> Three years ago, Jamie, a ward nurse, met Sheila, a medical resident, during the night shift in a city hospital. Shortly afterward, they began dating and a year later moved in together. Thereafter they had little sexual contact because, Jamie

said, she didn't like Sheila's sexual style. At the point of entering therapy, Jamie described herself as "completely turned off."

Because they pooled their money and friends, their differences in status and income were not evident on the surface. In response to the therapist's probing about these matters, Sheila stated that her overhead expenses—she started her own practice after her residency—made it difficult to ascertain her actual income, but, she said, it probably approximated Jamie's salary. The same measured, leveling responses met the therapist's queries about future opportunities, friends, and family. (The couple's difference in status and power was mirrored by their families of origin.)

The most striking thing about this passage is the therapist's insistent focus on income inequality. Even after the patients brought up their sexual interactions—after Jamie said she didn't like her partner's "sexual style" and, as a result, felt "completely turned off"—the therapist continued to direct the conversation to differences in status and power, a mode of response that seems unlike anything in case studies with heterosexuals.

The case study continued:

Whether deserved or not, the therapist said, doctors are venerated in our culture. They often have access to large incomes, prestige, and attention from both friends and strangers. Nurses, the therapist continued, are not accorded the same prestige and are, in fact, generally seen as much less than, and handmaidens to, doctors. It was important to look at the way this power difference affected each partner in the relationship.

After several more similar forays into the unmentionable by the therapist, Jamie was able to talk about some of her resentment. She said she could see Sheila basking in the attention she got from admiring friends at parties and it disgusted her. It wasn't unusual after these events for Sheila to want sex.

The surfacing of these differences and the accompanying resentment doesn't signal the partners' readiness for sex therapy exercises; it is simply one step in this direction. If the less powerful partner cannot replace sexual refusal with another power source of her own, either external or intrapsychic, it is unlikely that the imbalance in the bedroom can be corrected.[1]

It's possible, of course, that in this instance sex therapy focused on the partners' power and status differences, not because they are both women, but because of the therapist's unique theoretical interests. The fact remains, nonetheless, that I could not find any case studies with a comparable focus on power imbalances when the partners are a man and woman, while I did find several such cases in which the partners are both women. Consider, for example, this case study from the article, "Working with Same-Sex Couples" (Alonzo, 2005), which appeared in the *Handbook of Couple's Therapy*. That case study addressed the sexual problem of Sarah, aged forty-four, and her partner, Chris, aged twenty-nine. This lesbian couple had been together for two years when they began therapy at Sarah's insistence because she wanted more physical intimacy.[2] First, like the case of Jamie and Sheila, and unlike the case studies involving heterosexual partners, neither Chris nor Sarah was identified as mentally ill. Second, the therapy did not begin with discussions of the physiological and sensory dimensions of their sex life; there were no discussions of how the couple's sexual techniques or sexual machinery were in need of repair, and no discussions devoted to when and how the partners engaged in sex. What is most unusual about this case study, when contrasted with the treatment of heterosexual couples, is the immediate focus on socio-economic inequality, as if this same-sex couple's discrepancies in privilege and power were at least as significant as their discrepancies in sexual interest. In that regard, the therapist began by noting the partners' racial difference (Chris is black and Sarah is white) and that each partner has very different access to income, social privilege, and property, with Sarah owning the house they live in and having a substantially higher income as a realtor compared to Chris's earnings as a first grade teacher. The therapist left the question open as to how this inequality affected the couple's sex life, hypothesizing that perhaps Chris felt a need to reject Sarah's sexual overtures as a way of compensating for her perceived power deficit. But what appeared most unusual, as well as unmistakable, was the therapist's conviction that Chris and Sarah's therapy could not proceed without acknowledging that inequality and carefully considering its effects. This therapist, like Sheila's and Jamie's, treated socio-economic inequality as a foundational issue, affecting not only the couple's sexuality, but their entire relationship. "While the therapist must recognize Sarah's determination and diligence, the therapist must sensitively address the privileges that Sarah has that Chris does not—higher discretionary income, ownership of property, established professional status in the community, ability to be 'out' at work, and Caucasian status."[3]

Why this kind of focus is more likely to occur with same-sex, over opposite-sex partners—why socio-economic inequality may be easier to discuss—is not entirely clear. But because this kind of inequality is generally far greater between male and female partners than between members of the same sex—because "same sex couples," according to Lev and Nichols, "do not have the inherent imbalance that comes when two partners have been socialized differently and have unequal access to power in the world outside the marriage"[4]—that difference should be both easier to recognize among heterosexual couples and more consequential. Yet, for some reason, perhaps related to the fact that socio-economic inequality has so much bearing on the ways heterosexual partners interact, the topic is potentially more threatening to raise. In any case, it does not appear to factor into case studies involving heterosexual couples. Consider, for example, that in the cases from the chapter on "women's duty," in which women deferred to a husband's sexual wishes, sometimes making enormous sacrifices to give their man the sexual experience he wants, the question of their socio-economic inequality was not included in the case report. Consider that in the Kari–Greg case, Kari was willing to go through major surgery on her vagina in the hope of minimizing her pain during intercourse, because her husband, incorrectly, believed that her expressions of pain during intercourse indicated that she was not attracted to him. Why was Kari willing to do this for her husband? What was motivating her? In neither the Kari–Greg case, nor any of the other cases in that chapter, did the therapist examine the possibility, or indicate any suspicion, that a woman's decision to accede to her husband's sexual wishes, regardless of her sexual indifference, discomfort, and/or pain, might have something to do with his socio-economic power over her.

A Focus on the Relationship

Sam and Jo

The article "Emotionally Focused Therapy for Couples" (Grayer, 2016), which appeared in the journal, *Sexual and Relationship Therapy,* includes the case study of Sam, a woman who had breast cancer, which was treated with a lumpectomy, radiation, and long-term endocrine therapy. Sam's story reminded me of Mary, the woman in recovery from ovarian cancer who was discussed in the previous chapter. Both Sam and Mary were seen in sex therapy because of their inability to engage in sexual activity following their cancer treatments. Sam experienced a reduction in desire, while Mary became distressed during intercourse and could no longer achieve orgasm. In Mary's case, you might recall, she had undergone a total hysterectomy, an oophorectomy, and eight cycles of chemotherapy. But the major difference (apart from the fact that Mary, a heterosexual, was in her sixties, and Sam, a lesbian, was in her forties) was in their treatment. Sam was seen with her partner, Jo. Mary was seen alone, without her husband. Sam was not given a psychiatric diagnosis, while Mary was diagnosed with "female orgasmic disorder." And perhaps the most significant difference of all: in Sam's case, the therapy did not focus on getting her sexual functioning back on track with her partner, Jo. Instead, the emphasis was on understanding the personal meanings that loss of sexual interaction had for them.[5] By contrast, the exclusive focus in Mary's case was on her having intercourse and orgasm.

In therapy, Jo and Sam shared that one of the secondary consequences of Sam's loss of desire was her newly developed pattern of holding back from touching Jo in an affectionate way out of fear that those touches or hugs might stimulate Jo sexually, leading to sexual expectations that Sam did not feel she could deliver. Jo said that she interpreted the new physical difference between them as highly disturbing, mainly because, to her, it indicated that Sam no longer found her attractive and no longer loved her, not unlike the problems some men were said to have experienced in previous chapters. But unlike the heterosexual cases, Sam and Jo's problem was reframed as a relationship problem, specifically, a problem of feeling insecure in love, rather than a problem of physical sensation and sexual activity. In the therapist's words,

> it is important to help Sam and Jo become aware of their cycle of interaction together as early as possible. If the problem can be reframed as one that exists in the relationship, rather than located in either of them, it will be easier for them to come together as a team to look at the problem with curiosity and hope.[6]

Mary said that after her cancer treatments, what she missed most was the feeling of "closeness" she and her husband used to experience after intercourse. Nonetheless, this relationship problem was reframed as a problem of individual psychopathy. It was located inside her—hence her psychiatric diagnosis, female orgasmic disorder.

Liz and Scottie

To give one more example of how therapy with female couples focuses on the partnership over and above either partner's alleged psychiatric dysfunction, consider the case of a lesbian couple described in an article that appeared in the fourth edition of the *Principles and Practice of Sex Therapy*, "Therapy with Sexual Minorities" (Nichols and Schernoff, 2007). In this case, the couple, Liz and Scottie, both in their forties, began therapy because they said they were disappointed by the infrequency of their sexual relations, which occurred only once or twice a year. The therapist began the first session by asking them a question that rarely if ever appears in case studies involving heterosexual couples troubled by sexual disinterest. She asked "whether the couple genuinely wanted to be more sexual or whether they felt they were supposed to have more sex because sex was an indication of a healthy relationship."[7] This question shifted attention from the couple's sensory experiences and orgasms to the meaning of sexual activity and its role in their relationship. The therapist learned that Liz and Scottie's "problem," much like Sam and Jo's problem, was more emotional than sensual or physiological. Their initial reason for beginning sex therapy was Scottie's reaction to her discovery that Liz had been attracted to another woman. Scottie was frightened and insecure in their relationship, and her discomfort motivated her to seek couple's sex therapy as a way of preserving the relationship. In place of the conversation that so often occurs on sexual performance and responsiveness when the woman's sexually dissatisfied partner is a man, this therapist almost immediately turned the therapeutic conversation into a discussion of the partners' shared love and commitment. Instead of treatment focused on training and altering one partner to perform the kinds of sexual activities preferred by the other, lesbian couples' treatment, in cases like this one, tend to fashion the treatment goal as a flexible compromise. Liz had a greater need for orgasm than Scottie, who often had no interest in sex or orgasm but did enjoy caressing Liz. From these beginnings, they were able to redefine a sexual encounter "to include sensual/genital contact between them that may or may not result in orgasm for one or both partners, and if orgasm ensues, it may or may not be facilitated by one's partner."[8] The newly shaped relational dynamics also relieved the partners' sense of sexual obligation, making each responsible for her own orgasm (or absence thereof).

Externalizing the Problem

According to the article, "Multicontextual Sex Therapy with Lesbian Couples" (Iasenza, 2004), which appeared in *Quickies: The Handbook of Brief Sex Therapy*, Jan and Sue began therapy with the complaint of infrequent sexual activity and loss of sexual desire. They said that they last had sex eight months earlier and, before that, only about once a month. These long stretches without sex were all right with Jan, but not with Sue, who during the first therapy session accused Jan of being sexually indifferent to her. What should be noticed at this point is that, as in the study of Bill and his chronic fatigue in the chapter "Men's Free Will," the therapist in this study did not locate Jan and Sue's problem in one of the partners. Neither partner received a psychiatric diagnosis because the therapist externalized the problem. As she explained, "by locating the problem outside the couple, partners work together against the problem instead of against each other."[9]

The common problem for both to confront, in this instance, was identified as societal homophobia. In taking this couple's history, the therapist recognized that a major shift had occurred in their relationship four years earlier when Sue decided to attend a gay/lesbian AA group. She began making new friends who were openly gay, and these new friendships, coupled with Sue's intensified desire to come out more at home and at work, created tension with Jan, who wanted to remain closeted. The therapist helped them see that the beliefs, feelings, and behaviors that were causing their sexual difficulties were in fact by-products of something outside themselves—society's discrimination against homosexuals.

As in Bill's case, their conflict was not treated as a deficiency in them as individuals or as a couple. Sue and Jan's case also resembles Bill's in coming to a seemingly positive result: "Hearing this, Sue felt less angry with Jan, and Jan became less defensive. Both described their pain about growing up lesbian, feeling invisible in their families, and being rejected by loved ones who wouldn't accept their sexual orientation."[10] The therapist observed that Jan and Sue's experience of surviving as lesbians in a homophobic world had equipped them with a number of skills and strengths, including a greater appreciation of people's differences, sensitivity toward others' oppression, an awareness of social inequality and inequity, and an enhanced willingness to fight for social justice. The therapist made the point, also, that Jan's and Sue's appreciation of others' struggles was a resource they could use with each other "as they explored ways they might (or might not) choose to come out to friends, family, or coworkers."[11]

In addition to this strategy of externalizing the problem, this case, like the others involving lesbian couples, diverts sex therapy's laser focus on sexuality and sensory experience to an alternative focus on emotional and social dynamics, with a much greater concern for the couple's relationship as a whole. Thus, Jan and Sue's therapist paid particular attention to the ways Jan and Sue "began to share their needs, desires, and fears about coming out, deciding which people to jointly come out to, which to come out separately, and how to support each other in doing so."[12] As for their sex life, without any prompting from the therapist, the more they worked together at coming out, the more their sexual interest in each other seemed to resurface, as evidenced not so much in the frequency of sexual activity, as in the amount of thought and energy they devoted to it, for example, by co-authoring a sexual menu, which consisted of a list of their favorite sexual activities; watching woman-centered sex education films; and visiting erotic boutiques together.

This chapter asked whether sex therapy with lesbian couples, as described in the professional literature, is different from sex therapy with heterosexual couples. The conclusion, based on examination of published case studies, is that when both partners are women, sex therapy appears more attentive to the couple's relationship, more attentive to how sex fits into the relationship, how socioeconomic inequality affects their sexual interaction, the underlying *meanings* sex has for the partners, and the possibility of working out compromises. Along with those differences, when both partners are women, sex therapy appears less interested in applying psychiatric labels, less interested in training either or both partners to become better sexual technicians and performers, and less interested in singling out one of the partners as the one with problem—the one who has to change for the couple to resolve their sexual impasse.

10
Discontinuities, Deviations, and Reversals

> If after marriage, ability to enjoy intercourse completely and to attain release from orgasm is not achieved within a few weeks, seek expert advice. Do not let the wife form the habit of not enjoying it.
> —LeMon Clark, The Enjoyment of Love in Marriage (1969)

> The wife must be *taught*, not only how to achieve coitus, but, above all, how and what to feel in this unique act!
> —Theodor Van De Velde, Ideal Marriage (1926)

> Her duty is not only to have the sex she doesn't really want, but to enjoy it.
> —Germaine Greer, The Times (2003)

This book began with the story of the most overt type of repression: the story of a woman who was placed into a coma so her husband could copulate with her body at will. Now, I'd like to discuss cases that seem to reverse that kind of subjugation, cases where, in the name of treating a woman's sexual dysfunction, she isn't etherized, overpowered, or even pressured. Instead, she is taught how to become more attuned to her own feelings, to her own "authentic self." In other words, in this chapter, power operates more like a velvet glove than a mailed fist. Thus conceived, sex therapy discourse takes on the appearance of supporting a woman's autonomy and empowerment; it takes on the appearance of supporting her right to say "no" to her male partner's demands for sexual intercourse. The following examination of sex therapy case studies also reveals a hidden agenda wherein support for a woman's feelings and rights is accompanied by support for a man's right to be sexually demanding of her. The normal conclusion for these cases, paradoxically, is that the sexually resistant woman becomes less resistant and more compliant. What makes her more compliant may simply be the fact that, in these instances, power does not come down hard. It doesn't appear repressive. Saying "This is who you really are; this is what you need," works better than saying, "This is how you should behave; this is what you have to do."[1]

The Velvet Glove

Edward–Jocelyn

In "Strategic Treatment of Female Hypoactive Sexual Desire" (Pietsch, 2001), published in the peer-reviewed *Journal of Family Psychotherapy*, Edward, the husband, had threatened to leave his wife Jocelyn if she continued to refuse his sexual demands. As the therapist describes their interaction, Edward would begin by "asking Jocelyn for sexual intercourse, and her subsequent indirect refusal by avoiding him or not answering him directly with 'no,' initiated the sequence most of the time. He would become agitated and then she would become agitated. Edward would then . . . give his wife an unspecified threat that he was going to leave."[2]

Unlike other cases in which a sex therapist directly encourages the wife to become more sexually active and responsive by prescribing masturbation and sensate focus exercises, power, in this case study, operates in reverse; the therapist advises Jocelyn to say "no" whenever she doesn't want to have sex with Edward. The therapeutic method illustrated by this case encourages her to assert her sexual rights, a position that seems to directly contradict others surveyed in this collection.

For Foucault, the power of social control via the velvet glove comes from its invisibility, seamlessness, and ubiquity: "The judges of normality are everywhere. We are in the society of the teacher-judge, the doctor-judge, the educator-judge, the social-worker judge; it is on them that the universal reign of the normative is based."[3] For example, it's only upon closer inspection that we come to see that advising Jocelyn to say "no" to Edward was not intended to legitimate her sexual abstinence. Rather, it was intended to stimulate Jocelyn's sexual appetite, under the assumption that she would desire sex more if she felt she had the power to refuse: "The therapist pointed out that Jocelyn's overall goals of therapy were to increase her desire and sexual activity in their relationship, and get their marriage back on track. Consistently 'giving in' to sexual intercourse would not achieve those goals."[4]

According to the therapist, the strategy proved effective, because by the next session, "the frequency of intercourse had increased to three times over the past week." Two weeks later, Jocelyn "reported that the frequency of intercourse had increased, her husband was less grumpy, and she was happier."[5] Here's the paradox: in a case study in which the therapist explicitly sought to empower the female partner, the therapist expected the female partner to be the one to make the change. The therapist did not directly target for elimination the pressure Edward applied to Jocelyn to make her engage in intercourse. Only Jocelyn's reluctance to engage in intercourse—"female hypoactive desire disorder"—was identified as a problem. Moreover, progress was measured by a single standard, the same standard employed in almost all cases involving a woman's low sexual desire: the frequency of sexual activity. In this instance, the sex therapist appeared to regard the strategy of empowering Jocelyn as successful, not because she interpreted Jocelyn's supposed empowerment as an end in itself, but rather because it motivated Jocelyn to have intercourse more often, in a way that proved more satisfying to her male partner.

Anna–Derek

In another case study, this one from the journal, *Sexual and Relationship Therapy*, and titled, "Compassionate Authenticity: A Treatment Model for Working with Women with Low Libido" (Jernigan, 2014), the therapist similarly encourages a woman with low sexual interest to stand up for herself. This case involves Anna, aged twenty-four, who came to therapy with the complaint "that her marriage was falling apart because she did not want to have sex."[6] In her words, her husband Derek "wants it all the time, and I consent even though I don't want to."[7] Anna added that Derek is often "pushy," his sexual approach "felt intrusive," and he "had recently upped the ante by stating that he might leave the marriage because he felt unwanted, sexually." She summed up by saying that she hates sex. "But it makes him happy so I try."[8]

During the first phase of treatment, the therapist tried to help Anna become more in tune with her feelings—to listen "to the 'part' of her that quietly cried inside while having sex she did not want to have," to listen "to the 'part' of her that got angry on her own behalf and felt resentful and bitter towards her husband." Even though, as a result of these exercises, Anna began to feel at peace with saying "no" to Derek's sexual advances, even though she began to "see her sexual withdrawal as an understandable and adaptive response to unwanted sexual contact,"[9] the therapist did not see this as an appropriate stopping point. As in Jocelyn's case, Anna's therapist wanted Anna to eventually come around to saying "yes" to her husband's sexual advances. As a result, the therapy that began with the explicit goal of authorizing and validating a woman's right to resist her male partner's sexual demands reverted to the more traditional sex therapy technique of erotic touching exercises for the partners. According to the therapist, this approach "helped Anna make space for her authentic sensual self."[10] This was followed by another erotic exercise, in which the therapist asked Anna to go home and blindfold Derek, tie his hands together, and then do "whatever she wanted" to his body. According to Anna, the exercise proved extremely successful: "it was like a switch got flipped; I started out a bit tentative, and then at some point something changed and I was *really* into it. Derek was pretty psyched, too!" At the conclusion of treatment, the therapist described Anna's progress this way: "Her libido is active, she enjoys her sensuality, and when she chooses to, she shares it with her husband on her terms."[11]

It may well be that Jocelyn and Anna wanted to learn to enjoy sex with their husbands, and it may well be that they did learn to enjoy it "on their terms." However, it's also possible that the therapist overlooked two other contingencies: Jocelyn and Anna may have needed help learning that's it okay to dislike sex. They may have needed help learning how to live with a sexually demanding man without feeling that the only option available to them is to become more sexually active and responsive. In both the Jocelyn–Edward and Anna–Derek cases, it's possible that, instead of focusing on awakening a woman's sexual responsiveness to her husband, the therapist could have chosen to focus on awakening the husband's responsiveness to his wife's nonsexual virtues. Instead of focusing on changing a woman who had been the object of sexual bullying, the therapist could have focused on changing the bully.

Patricia–Edward

The case study, "Sexual Interest/Arousal Disorder in Women" (Brotto and Luria, 2014), appeared in the fifth edition of the *Principles and Practice of Sex Therapy*, and concerns Patricia, a forty-eight-year-old teacher and her husband, Edward, who "presented for treatment after struggling with discrepant desire in their relationship for the full duration of their 15-year marriage."[12] The authors specified that, like most heterosexual couples with a discrepancy in sexual interest, the man wanted more sex and the woman wanted less. In Patricia's case, she "rarely experienced any erotic thoughts," "had difficulty identifying any triggers for her sexual desire or response," found "sex occasionally painful due to lack of lubrication," "could not identify non-genital signs of arousal within her body," "had never experienced a pronounced sexual response or sexual pleasure in the past," "had a very low interest in sexual activity for her entire life," and "her motivations for sex stemmed primarily from a need to keep Edward happy, even though she derived no personal satisfaction out of sex."[13] Edward, for his part, had "declared that he could not envision himself remaining in this relationship if Patricia's sexual difficulties did not improve."[14] The proposed solution, according to the authors, consisted of heightening Patricia's awareness of her body and mind:

> Patricia was introduced to mindfulness skills, initially for up to 10 minutes in a session and subsequently 30 minutes daily practice of her body scan at home. She was encouraged to suspend any attachment toward needing to be "fixed" but, rather, to be with her moment-to-moment sensations. After a period of

weeks, this allowed Patricia to identify body sensations that were experienced as positive, and her practice also allowed her to explore her anxiety more fully in a compassionate and nonjudgmental manner. She learned that from her earliest interactions, sex had been quite stressful to her, due to having partners who blamed her for not reaching orgasm.[15]

As Patricia became more self-aware, her treatment was extended, like Anna's, to include sexual exercises. Also, like Anna's therapy experience, as far as we can tell from the case study, Paula's sexual exercises worked out fairly well:

Edward responded positively to Patricia's newfound response and therefore began to initiate nonintercourse sexual encounters more often. The introduction of sensate focus exercises then encouraged Patricia to verbalize what she experienced as pleasure to Edward. By the end of 1 year of treatment, Patricia felt that she had gained some interest in sexual activity, was fully aware of the responsive nature of sexual desire, and found their sexual interactions to be pleasurable.[16]

It's hard to overlook the guarded language. What does it mean to say that Patricia's sexual exercises encouraged her to "verbalize what she experienced as pleasure to Edward"? Does it mean that she actually learned to take pleasure in her sexual activities, or does it mean that she only learned to "verbalize" pleasure? What does it mean to say that, after a year of treatment, "Patricia felt that she had gained some interest in sexual activity" and "was fully aware of the responsive nature of sexuality"? Does it mean that she was now interested in engaging in sexual activity, or does it mean that she had simply become interested in the topic of sexuality and its "responsive nature"? Does it mean she developed the capacity to become sexually responsive or had she merely learned how to "'be natural' and play the part?"

We will never know for sure. What we can say is that the text gives no evidence that Patricia's therapist had any suspicion that Patricia, a woman who had never shown any interest in sex, but now says she wants, more than anything, to preserve her marriage, might engage in "information management." She might have fabricated the kinds of responses most likely to make her husband happy and ensure the survival of her marriage. All we can say about Patricia's case, or Jocelyn's, or Anna's, is that they all follow the same narrative trajectory of therapeutic success: a woman who initially had experienced sex as aversive finally has a positive sexual experience with her husband at the end. The therapists do not appear to consider other possible trajectories: positive sexual experience is the desired outcome from the beginning. Within the profession, the rationale for this narrative exclusivity has a long history stretching back through Masters and Johnson to

Dora and Freud: the belief that we are all innately sexual and that we all have a fundamental capacity to enjoy intercourse and orgasm. If some, like Jocelyn, Anna, and Patricia, find that they can't enjoy intercourse and orgasm, this absence of pleasure in sex must stem from some kind of personal anxiety or fear blocking the way. Somewhere along the way, they must have learned to fear their sexual potential. This line of reasoning may explain why the therapists involved in these cases appeared to see their job not as coercion, but as liberation—freeing women from neurotic or pathological inhibitions and helping them connect to their authentic, yet latent, sexual energies.

Training Her Softly

The next case study ("Getting in the Mood [for a Change]: Stage Appropriate Clinical Work for Sexual Problems"; Miller et al., 2004, published in *Quickies: The Handbook of Brief Sex Therapy*) appears to advocate a more positive and equitable therapeutic approach than most because of the therapist's remarkable patience and understanding. The woman in this case, like many other wives described in this survey, wanted to solve her intercourse problem for the sake of her husband's pleasure: "I don't expect to enjoy it but if I can just do it, it would satisfy Tom. As long as it doesn't hurt, I'll be satisfied."[17] Unlike the therapists in many of those other cases, however, this therapist makes a point of "going slow." She did not ask Francis to stretch her vagina with dilators. Nor did she ask Francis to imagine that she had a cavernous vagina easily capable of accommodating her husband's penis. Instead, Francis was instructed to limit herself to inserting Q-tips into her vagina. The rationale for beginning this way she explained as follows:

> Overall, it is respectful to show the understanding that change requires time, thoughtfulness, and sometimes radical accommodation. Helping take the pressure off, a therapist adopting such a position gives clients the space and support to commit to change.[18]

If the therapist had told Francis to insert a dilator into her vagina, Francis might have balked. A smaller insert, such as a Q-tip, is less threatening. With a Q-tip, a woman in training for intercourse is not only less likely to resist, her therapist is less likely to feel or appear coercive. The therapist, in this instance, does indeed seem humane and understanding, showing remarkable respect for her female patient's resistance and thereby deflecting accusations of sexism or misogyny. Despite the gentle approach, however, the engine driving this therapy is the man's needs for sex and for affirmation of his sexual attractiveness. The woman's pleasure in the relationship is more or less irrelevant to the female partner ("I don't expect to enjoy it"), a position that went unchallenged by the therapist. The pace of change was slower, and the objects inserted into her vagina were smaller, but the goal was the same: to make Francis more receptive to the intercourse her husband needed to find pleasure in the relationship.

Foregrounding the Relationship

The approach illustrated by the next case study ("Using Emotionally Focused Therapy to Treat Sexual Desire Discrepancy in Couples"; Girard and Wooley, 2017, from the *Journal of Sex & Marital Therapy*), also appears more positive and equitable than most because of the therapist's explicit effort to shift the therapeutic focus away from the woman's sexual disinterest. Unlike other sex therapy interventions involving heterosexuals, this one doesn't have a designated patient; no one received a psychiatric diagnosis. Instead, therapy was directed to both partners, to their relationship—specifically, to the discrepancy between their levels of sexual interest. As the therapist explained,

> shifting the perspective from one partner's low desire to sexual desire discrepancy moves the diagnostic and therapeutic process from the individual to the dyadic level and creates a space for the individual with lower desire to be viewed within the context of the relationship, rather than pathologized or seen as dysfunctional.[19]

This kind of reframing is entirely in keeping with Tiefer's recommendations for feminist sex therapy[20] and is obviously an improvement over the kind of gender imbalance implicitly endorsed in the treatment of women who were held solely responsible for the couple's sexual problem. But does this reframe ultimately succeed in placing the woman's sexual interests on the same plane as the man's? Does the shift in the therapeutic focus from the individual to the dyad mean that the woman's professed dislike of sex is treated with the same respect as the man's professed need for sex?[21]

In this case, a heterosexual couple, Adam and Jen had been living together for about a year when they separated "due to issues with lack of intimacy and sexual frequency."[22] The separation lasted only a month, but after they resumed living together, their sexual problems continued. Jen did not desire Adam sexually; "she felt pressured to have sex and would otherwise not think about it at all," and her sexual disinterest made Adam feel "extremely stressed."[23] They had frequent arguments about the lack of sexual activity, and, like several of the men in the cases discussed in previous chapters, "Adam got angry and threatened to leave Jen if she did not fix this part of the relationship."[24] The authors did not say whether Adam initiated their separation, but it's likely that he did, since the reasons for that separation ("lack of intimacy and sexual frequency") are the same reasons he gave for his continuing threats to separate. His threats to separate, in other words, had a long history, and must have felt very real to Jen since he had a record of acting on them.

Also consistent with the other cases, Adam's extortion made matters worse. Jen attempted to comply with his sexual demands, but the pressure to perform only increased her anxiety and sense of defeat. As she told Adam during one of their therapy sessions, "I feel like I can't make you happy, and that eventually you are going to leave me. I'm terrified of losing you."[25]

A third commonality is that the power differential between the partners, which perhaps made it possible for the man to threaten the woman, was not discussed or acknowledged. Instead, the therapy centered on Adam's and Jen's feelings. According to the study's authors, "the focus was on owning and sharing their deeper fears.... For Adam, these fears were focused on his view of himself as being unwanted and rejected. Jen's underlying fear surrounded her feeling not good enough and defective."[26]

The authors justify devoting so much time and attention to the couple's emotions because their goal, as they explained it, was to help the couple "connect emotionally, thereby increasing the desire for physical connection."[27] Simply put, the authors hoped that helping the partners share their deepest feelings would motivate them to have sex with each other. But, significantly, Adam never had a "problem" with his sexual motivation. He always desired physical connection with Jen. In fact, his main complaint about Jen was that she didn't want sex. Her failure to experience and express a similar kind and level of desire is what brought them to therapy in the first place. Yet somehow, in this case study's rhetoric—"in shifting the perspective from one partner's low desire to sexual discrepancy"— Jen's issue, her low sexual desire, became reformulated as the couple's shared issue. Despite the shift in language from the individual to the dyad, once again, only the woman was expected to change, and the kind of change expected of her was the same kind of change routinely charted as therapeutic success in women who begin sex therapy in response to their male partner's threats. The way to achieve the common goal of continuing the relationship was to make the woman more sexually open and available to her partner. Even though "Jen continued to report lower spontaneous desire in session," her therapist reported that as treatment progressed, "she was more open to being sexually intimate."[28]

In the case as presented, the therapist did not identify Adam's threats to leave as problematic, despite the fact that he made them repeatedly, they had a devastating effect on Jen, and they were subject to Adam's conscious control. He could have stopped threatening to leave if he so decided, and the therapist might reasonably have made this suggestion. But only Jen's lack of desire was targeted for change, even though it was not subject to her control. She wanted to desire Adam sexually, she wanted to enjoy sexual intercourse with him, but it was beyond her power. She could not make herself respond to Adam in the ways Adam wanted. The therapist could have asked Adam if he could reconcile himself to this fact—that Jen wanted to desire him, but for the time being, could not make herself. The therapist could have asked Adam to consider the possibility that Jen might prefer a close but asexual relationship. The therapist could have also asked Adam if he could focus more on the good things he had with Jen, rather than dwell on what he did not have. But according to the case description, those issues were not explored. Instead, the therapist recommended that Adam and Jen practice low-key sexual activities at home such as sensual touch and sensate focus exercises, the kind designed by Masters and Johnson to release sexual desire—to "free sexual dysfunctional individuals from inhibitions that deprive them of an opportunity to respond naturally to sensory experience."[29]

These exercises may have been prescribed for both partners, but they were in fact for the benefit of only one of the partners, the one who wanted more sex—the man. Like the therapist who recommended that Francis insert Q-tips into her vagina, Jen and Adam's therapist had a more humane, more feminist-appearing approach, but the goal appeared the same as for the "wife" whose vagina was stretched with dilators: to get the woman to conform to the man's sexual agenda —to make her more sexually responsive and accommodating.

Giving Women a Voice

In 1994, in recognition that many people with little sexual interest manage to lead comfortable and successful lives, the American Psychiatric Association stipulated that before a woman with little sexual interest could be diagnosed with a psychiatric disorder, she had to claim she was markedly distressed by her lack of interest in sex. The distress criterion was retained for the *DSM-5* (2013),[30] largely because it seemed more empowering for women to decide for themselves, rather than to have a clinician decide for them, that their low sexual interest represents a significantly distressing problem.[31] A sex therapy case that appeared in the *DSM-Clinical Cases* (2014), a volume written to specify and demonstrate *DSM-5* diagnoses, tests whether the "distress criterion" has changed anything. Does the insistence on this criterion indeed help empower female patients in sex therapy, or does the long-standing bias in favor of men still prevail?[32]

Elizabeth, a successful attorney in her late thirties, originally presented for couples counseling because of increased bickering with Finn, her fiancé. When the therapist met with Finn, also an attorney in his late thirties, he said that the couple's biggest problem was Elizabeth's disinterest in sex. "She seemed to go through the motions, he said, and always relied on alcohol."[33] He said that before they could have sex, she needed to get drunk. However, in the therapist's meeting with Elizabeth, Elizabeth provided a very different account. She said she found her partner too sexually demanding: "As it was, he wanted sex every time they got together, often twice in the same night." Elizabeth identified his demanding behavior as her reason for getting drunk before she had sex—to numb herself. "Although alcohol made intercourse acceptable," she said, "'arousal was almost never tolerable.'"[34] She also said she would have broken up with Finn because of his demandingness, but decided to stay the course because she was nearing forty and believed this might be her last chance to have children. While the *DSM-Clinical Cases* concluded that Elizabeth's life-long sexual disinterest indicated the "possibility of female sexual interest/desire disorder" and "warranted further exploration," no definitive diagnosis was made. The reason: Elizabeth did not communicate personal distress about her own sexuality. Rather, she only communicated distress about her partner's sexual demandingness—his insistence on making sex a central part of their relationship. From a feminist perspective, this represents a positive development. By appealing to the personal distress criterion for the diagnosis of "female sexual interest/arousal disorder," the male partner's complaint didn't succeed in becoming the final word on how to judge Elizabeth's sexuality. Elizabeth wasn't silenced, nor was she pressured to accommodate her male partner's sexual needs.

At the same time, we should probably hesitate before asserting that Elizabeth was treated in a gender-neutral, egalitarian way, considering that the entire case study is intended to illustrate the profession's response to the question of how to apply a psychiatric diagnosis to a woman who refuses to comply with a man's sexual demands. The entire case, in other words, is devoted to sifting through the available evidence to confirm or disconfirm the possibility of Elizabeth's "female sexual interest/arousal disorder" diagnosis. Whether Elizabeth was ultimately found to be abnormal or normal, she is featured in this case as potentially dysfunctional/mentally ill—potentially pathological—although she herself never complained about any dimension of her sexual behavior or psychological status. The only complaints about Elizabeth came from her male partner, Finn. While her complaints about him appeared as numerous and intense as his about her, he, unlike Elizabeth, at no point comes under consideration as a candidate for psychiatric diagnosis.

Obviously, this couple had a sexual incompatibility issue: their sexual needs were almost diametrically opposed. But somehow, in this case study, once again, only the female partner's sexual history and sexual needs (or lack thereof), come under surveillance as fundamentally problematic. The intense psychiatric scrutiny directed at Elizabeth but not at her male partner suggests that the kinds of pro-male, anti-female biases inherited from the previous century, far from having been rooted out of the diagnosis and treatment of low sexual interest, remain intact, but in a somewhat different, less explicit form. Elizabeth was not, in the end, diagnosed, nor was she pressured to accommodate her partner's sexual needs, but she was always subject to psychiatric scrutiny. That the sexual dysfunction in this case was discussed and assessed as Elizabeth's alone, and not as a problem shared by her partner, suggests that if she and her partner were to continue their treatment, she would have been the only one expected to change. She would have been expected to desire sex more, with no comparable expectation for her partner. It is also likely that many other women in Elizabeth's shoes would have blamed themselves for their male partner's frustration. They would have felt there was something wrong with themselves for not satisfying their man in the way our culture teaches us that men, particularly men in the husband or fiancé role, deserve to be sexually satisfied.[35] Without openly acknowledging that they were deferring to their man's needs, these women might have attempted to persuade themselves, their male partner, and their therapist, that they were indeed "markedly distressed" by their low sexual interest and arousal when in fact they might simply be distressed by their partner's distress. Said differently, they might have deferred to the man's needs not because he, or anyone else, applies direct pressure and not because he insists, but because they believe that deference is appropriate.

The problem here, as Hare-Mustin explained, is that women's deference to men, even when it feels reasonable and freely chosen, is still deference. "Acceptable masculinity is still domination."[36]

Conclusion

> The primary suggestion I can make at this point is the perennial feminist one: Challenge all assumptions; reexamine everything. Once you remember that sex research is fundamentally political, fundamentally about power, you will be better prepared for the long haul.
> —Leonore Tiefer, "Feminist Critique of Sex Therapy"

Psychiatrists, psychologists, and sex therapists of all kinds want to confront and alleviate women's sexual problems. Whether the sexual problems center on pain during intercourse such as "genito-pelvic pain/penetration disorder," or involuntary spasms or contractions such as "vaginismus," or center on the absence of desire such as "inhibited sexual desire disorder," "aversive sexual desire disorder, "female orgasmic disorder," "hypoactive sexual desire disorder," or "sexual interest/arousal disorder," therapists treat these conditions as pre-existing, objective realities that may require elaborate, costly, and sometimes painful treatments.

Yet, it is often difficult to say whether these diagnoses are actually helping, and in fact, it is difficult to pinpoint what these diagnoses actually mean. There is so much variability in women's sexual responses, especially given their connection to the emotional aspects of a relationship, that the concepts, "normal" and "abnormal," seem almost incomprehensible.[1] What makes a sexual pattern or condition a psychiatric disorder? The question is particularly relevant to low sexual interest, the most common sexual dysfunction among women. Most of us, at some (or many) points in our lives, feel relatively indifferent to sex. Maybe we're too tired, or we're preoccupied with other things, or we don't feel particularly attracted to anyone. The point is that sexual indifference is not really very rare.[2] And if it's not rare, what makes it abnormal?

According to the *DSM-5*, distress is the key. If a woman suffers distress because of her low sexual interest, she may be diagnosed with a psychiatric disorder. The problem with using the distress criterion, however, is that many conditions cause distress that are not usually classified as mental illness. Take pregnancy and childbirth, for example. It would be absurd to call pregnancy or childbirth a psychiatric disorder simply because it's associated with distress. Another problem is that the *DSM-5* identifies several conditions as psychiatric disorders, such as narcissistic personality disorder, which have no association with feelings of distress. To give one more reason why feelings of distress are unsatisfactory markers of mental illness, the *DSM-5* noted that a woman may experience distress in combination with low sexual interest, but her distress may be more closely related to her partner's negative reactions to her lack of sexual interest than to her own reactions to that condition. Thus, the *DSM-5* stipulated that "if interpersonal or significant cultural factors, such as severe relationship distress, intimate partner violence, or other significant stressors explain sexual interest/arousal symptoms, then a diagnosis of sexual interest/arousal disorder would not be made."[3] If a woman's partner is abusive to her because she has been unwilling to sleep with him, it makes no sense to say she has a psychiatric disorder. It would probably make more sense to say the abusive partner is the one with the psychiatric disorder.

A second quality commonly associated with the mental illness/psychiatric disorder label is impaired functioning. Assuming this criterion, we might be able to say that a woman who dislikes sex can be said to have a psychiatric disorder because she's missing out on an important life experience. However, the "impaired functioning criterion" has problems too. Imagine saying, for example, that people who prefer to travel in their home country, rather than go abroad, are mentally ill since they're missing out on another important life experience. The problem here, of course, is that, by following this logic, the definition of a "psychiatric disorder" can expand endlessly or can be keyed to culturally dictated notions of what is "normal" behavior. What's to prevent someone from arguing that people who prefer to remain childless or refuse to purchase a smart phone or install air conditioning, by limiting their horizons so severely, must be mentally ill? Robert L. Spitzer, the leader of the American Psychiatric Association task force responsible for reformulating the *DSM-III*, the first edition to include "inhibited sexual desire" as a psychiatric disorder, argued that the question of what is and is not an important life experience is actually critical to the question of what is and is not a psychiatric disorder. He offered this imaginary dialogue with a shoe fetishist to illustrate his point:

FETISHIST: Why is my preference for women's shoes a mental disorder?
SPITZER: You must admit that your behavior is extremely atypical. Hardly anyone needs women's shoes to be turned on.
FETISHIST: Certainly you are not using a statistical concept of normality; otherwise, you would have to classify genius as pathology.
SPITZER: You have a point there. However, from the evolutionary point of view, if all individuals had your condition, the human race would die out.
FETISHIST: But I understand that your APA has decided that homosexuality itself is not a mental disorder, so certainly you cannot use that argument. And if everyone were a psychiatrist, we would also be in big trouble.

SPITZER: Well, maybe it comes down to our view that certain critical life experiences and inner conflicts explain your behavior.
FETISHIST: I am sure that is correct, but I understand that all behavior, including your sexual preferences, whatever they are, are also determined by your life experiences and the way you have resolved your inner conflicts. I am beginning to think that there is something about my preference itself that your profession doesn't care for.
SPITZER: Well, I think you may have hit on something there. We do believe that optimal sexual functioning involves two human beings (at least) and not exclusively or preferentially inanimate objects.
FETISHIST: Why do you believe that?
SPITZER: I guess we believe that if you are unable to be sexually aroused by another human being you are at a disadvantage.
FETISHIST: Why is it a disadvantage? Shoes are easy to get.
SPITZER: I guess that deep in our bones we must believe that sex is more fulfilling when it is between human beings.
FETISHIST: That doesn't sound like a scientific fact but only your value judgment.[4]

What Spitzer's imaginary dialogue demonstrates is that the diagnosis of "psychiatric disorder" always involves a value judgment. And since women, according to the literature, are much more likely than men to be diagnosed with low sexual desire, with an estimated prevalence rate of thirty to fifty-five percent,[5] the judgment that a woman's lack of sexual interest is pathological appears to value men's sexuality over women's, leading to the conclusion that women should be more like men. Psychiatrists like Spitzer in his dialogue seem to believe "deep in their bones" that women should want sex as much as men want it. Moreover, they seem to believe that women should want it the way men want it, with intercourse leading to orgasm. This professional bias probably explains why the sex therapists examined in this book seemed to assume that the wives who did not want to have sex with their husbands would be better off if they could come around to desiring them. These therapists seemed to assume that it is unreasonable to ask a man, irrespective of his partner's disinterest, revulsion, or pain, to live without sex. And they seemed to assume the corollary position, that a woman can and should match her male partner's level of sexual desire and activity, despite all the evidence that a woman's sexuality is different than a man's, especially with regard to the frequency of desire, with all the research concurring that she is the one most likely to be saying, or thinking, "Not tonight, dear."[6]

Imposing a male model of sexuality onto women will obviously interfere with their ability to enjoy sex, as well as with their ability to maintain the psychological and emotional quality of their lives. What is somewhat less obvious is that these same psychiatric labels and treatments hurt men too. It's not only that in all the iterations of the *DSM*, a heterosexual man has been required, as a condition of his psychiatric health, to thrust his hard penis into a vagina and that failure to hold off ejaculation for at "approximately one minute" will turn him into a "premature ejaculator"[7]; it's that these rigid rules interfere with men's capacity to get close to their partners; they interfere with men's capacity to experience intimacy, to know their partners as persons.[8]

In the sex therapy case studies examined here, the "essentialist" assumption of an innate sexual drive complements the belief that women should respond to men's sexual advances with compliance and pleasure. The two complement one another because the notion of a natural inborn sexual drive, which seeks the continuous release of sexual energy, has clarified for therapists, as well as for the frustrated male and his noncompliant female partner, who is responsible for the problem—the female. She is the one blocking the flow of the couple's sexual energy. Thus, when heterosexual couples seek therapy for a discrepancy in sexual interest, when the woman desires little or no sexual activity and the man wants more, the woman is the one expected to change.[9] The problem with this is self-evident: endorsing a woman's right to sexual pleasure can be emancipatory, but requiring her to express sexual pleasure in particular ways under particular circumstances is just another way to compromise her autonomy. Sex therapists may reject conversion/reparative therapy for gay people, believing that therapy aimed at converting homosexuals into heterosexuals "may cause irreparable psychological, emotional, and spiritual harm,"[10] but the sex therapists in case studies presented as exemplary professional practice seem to show no comparable hesitancy when attempting to convert women who experience no sexual attraction into women who do.

How does a woman tainted with the stigma of low sexual desire respond? In the cases examined here, women seemed to make a sincere attempt to correct their alleged failing. They appeared to follow the sex therapist's instructions, and in most instances, they, along with their male partners, soon claimed that the problem that brought the couple to therapy, most commonly, the woman's lack of sexual interest, has either disappeared, or has progressed in the desired direction. She soon claimed to be experiencing at least some of the responses her therapist and male partner expect of her, all of which seems to support the notion that the way the superordinate class (men), expects the subordinate class (women) to behave does in fact affect how that class behaves, or claims to behave—a self-fulfilling expectation: Women actually arrange their lives to affirm what men want to see. We can call this "women's socialization" or "men's privilege and power," but in sex therapy, it is barely perceptible as a process. For the most part, women's sexual compliance appears voluntary, a matter of their free will. However, in her book, *Feminism Unmodified*, Catharine MacKinnon argues that "free will" has nothing to do with it:

> What I'm saying is, men's power to *make* the world here is their power to make us make the world of their sexual interaction with us the way they want it. They want us to have orgasms; that proves they're virile, potent, effective. We provide them that appearance, whether it's real for us or not. We even get into it. Our reality is, it is far less damaging and dangerous for us to do this, to accept a lifetime of simulated satisfaction, than to hold out for the real thing from them.[11]

At this point, perhaps we can agree that there is always the possibility that a woman in treatment for disliking sex might be engaged in "information management," given the association between low desire and mental illness. There is always the concern that a woman reporting on sexual desire might be trying to pass as someone she is not to remove the opprobrium of psychiatric disorder, and possibly the threat of losing her marriage, her home, and financial support. In either case, whether a woman in treatment for low sexual desire genuinely changes or only creates the appearance of genuinely changing, a basic contingency in these cases is stigma and social pressure. The psychiatric diagnosis for women's low sexual interest may not have been designed to extort women's sexual conformity, but that may be how it works. In Erving Goffman's words, "because of the great rewards in being considered normal, almost all persons who are in a position to pass will do so on some occasion by intent."[12]

If we want people to speak honestly about their low sexual desire, the solution appears obvious: we need to remove the stigma from low sexual desire, along with the other penalties that our culture routinely places on it. As C. J. Chasin argued in her article, "Reconsidering Asexuality and Its Radical Potential," we also need to interrogate the expectation that people, especially women, should want more sexual desire; we need to challenge the idea that sexual desire, in and of itself, is something to be valued. If it's okay for asexual people to not want sex, then why shouldn't it be okay for anyone to not want sex. Why can't we have a world without sanctions for not wanting sex? And why can't we have a world where being sexual is not a prerequisite of normalcy or intimacy?[13]

How Does Sex Therapy Survive?

The gender biases revealed by an analysis of case studies that serve to codify sex therapy methods and understandings appear to support men's sexual interests over women's sexual interests. And this brings us to an important puzzle, the question of how and why these biases survive.

To address that question, we need to first recognize that this problem goes far beyond sex therapy. We need to consider that pro-male bias infuses the sexual norms and expectations of Western culture, in general, including the sexual norms and expectations that women patients bring to sex therapy. As evidenced in several of the cases examined here, women may feel anxious about their perceived obligation to copulate with their male partners, but instead of regarding that sense of obligation as the problem, they, along with their husbands and therapists, may interpret women's anxiety as *the* problem. Women may blame themselves rather than identify their anxiety as a response to non-violent sexual coercion. This is how victims of violent sexual coercion respond, according to a recent volume on sexual violence in marriage: "The silence, blame, and/or shame associated with marital rape mean that few survivors of marital rape voluntarily self-disclose."[14] With regard to women patients in sex therapy, as far as we can tell from the review of exemplary training cases, women find little or no encouragement to speak out against unwanted, unpleasurable intercourse or to assert their right to desire as much or as little sexual activity as they want; instead, they are encouraged to adapt to their man's sexual needs.

For sex therapists who wish to overcome "himpathy" and give each patient the same kind of respect, regardless of gender, the problem posed by women's silence, self-blame, and denial appears obvious. Nothing could be more difficult (and awkward) for a sex therapist than trying recognize, or even imagine, a man as sexually coercive, when he is sitting in the therapist's office, and perhaps paying the therapist's fees, with his wife beside him, perhaps holding his hand, saying that she wants nothing more than to learn to become more sexually responsive and pleasing to him. Nothing could be more difficult than recognizing someone as sexually coercive when his wife, and everyone else, is saying he is not.

If sex therapy, as an institution, has been biased in favor of men, it is not alone in this bias. Many other Western institutions, such as household labor, workplace compensation, and childcare, have also been biased in favor of men. Sex therapy represents only one brick in the institutional edifice of male privilege that justifies, rationalizes, and normalizes male dominance in sexual, as well as in other male–female relational dynamics. When a sex therapist teaches a woman how to accept her husband's penis into her vagina, even though the woman dreads the idea—when a therapist encourages a woman to view her "other third shift" as healthful, personally rewarding, and socially necessary, regardless of her own needs and preferences—the unintended effect is "another brick in the wall" of a civil order devoted to male supremacy.

Sex therapy's link to pro-male ideology may survive not only because it assumes the mantle of "patriarchal truth" but also because it assumes the mantle of "scientific truth." It survives in large part because its arguments and techniques are framed as the product of impartial, objective research such as the case studies published in sex therapy journals and textbooks. And it survives because it does not operate alone. Sex therapy works through systems of mutually re-enforcing norms, disciplines, meanings, and tactics, many of which, when examined in isolation, appear too petty to notice. In Foucault's words, "these are humble modalities, minor procedures, as compared with the majestic rituals of sovereignty of the great apparatuses of state"[15] But when these "minor procedures" are taken together, they have the power of a grand strategy.

To borrow a metaphor from Marilyn Frye, if we look at only one wire of a birdcage up close, we may not be able to understand how it succeeds in keeping a bird from flying away. If we focus myopically on that one wire, it does not seem to have much deterrent power. But if we step back a bit and take in the larger picture, we can see how the cage wires intersect.[16] Considering the connections between sex therapy and other social institutions brings the cage into focus, making it clear that, although the details vary from woman to woman and from couple to couple, what women experience in sex and in sex therapy with their male partners may not be entirely different from women's experience in their other service roles. As a rule, the context in which women's service takes place, whatever the nature of that service, is one in which men have greater social, economic, political, and physical power than women. As a result of men's greater power, women are held responsible, and learn to hold themselves responsible, for good outcomes for men, more than men hold themselves responsible, or are held responsible, for good outcomes for women. Also, as a result of men's greater power, women's service work, as represented in female-dominated jobs such as prostitute, maid, cook, house cleaner, receptionist, administrative assistant, childcare worker, nurse's aide, nurse, wife, and mother, generally entails personal service, including sexual service (providing for men's sexual needs, bearing their children, "looking nice," wearing makeup, and "dressing attractively"), and ego service (providing men with admiration, support, and attention).[17] Of course, social power comes from sources other than male privilege—for example, wealth and wisdom. Accordingly, some women can be said to have more power than some men. By the same token, however, Dworkin notes that "all men have some kinds of power over all women; and most men have controlling power over what they call *their* women—the women they fuck. The power is predetermined by gender, by being male."[18]

Can Sex Therapy Change?

In the 1850s, a physician encountered no opposition to putting a woman into a coma so that her husband could copulate with her on demand. The only thing the physician required from the wife was her compliant vagina, a point of view that, in some ways, persists to this day. In none of the cases reviewed did a sex therapist advise a husband to accept that his wife could not become more sexually responsive to him While I did find therapists who advised a woman to accept her husband's sexual disinterest, as well as therapists who advised a woman to accept her lesbian partner's sexual disinterest, in my research for this book, I looked for, but did not find, case studies in which a therapist attempted to help a husband become more attuned to his wife's need to free herself from the obligation to please him sexually. What I found instead are cases in which the therapist tried to help the wife match her husband's level of sexual need. The husband's sexual drive always stood as the standard to which his wife should conform.

In recent years, while the field of psychotherapy has grown increasingly interested in the problems of child sexual abuse and violent spousal abuse, it has largely overlooked the role of sexual coercion in patients' and couples' ongoing, committed relationships. We have had little systematic study of sexual violence in marriage,[19] only a handful of studies on nonviolent sexual coercion among unmarried college students,[20] and still fewer studies on nonviolent sexual coercion among married couples.[21] Feminist critics of sex therapy, although concerned about male dominance and privilege in marriage, only briefly allude to nonviolent sexual coercion as a marital problem. The #MeToo movement may have prompted an ongoing public conversation about coercion in the forms of sexual harassment and assault committed by high-profile bosses and celebrities, but, to date, an analogous concern has not entered the public conversation for domestic coercion, as long-tern committed relationships have been pretty much off the #MeToo radar.

Feminist critics have explained this silence as a sign of our cultural belief that violent sexual coercion sets the standard for determining sexual abuse,[22] so that any coercion falling short of physically overwhelming a woman is not usually seen as serious.[23] This standard not only obscures the experiences of women who show signs of nonviolent sexual coercion, including the experiences of most female patients in sex therapy[24] it also trivialize those experiences as psychologically insignificant. When a man holds a knife to a woman's throat to obtain her sexual cooperation, sexual coercion is obvious, and we have no difficulty calling it rape. But when a nonviolent husband's demand for sexual intercourse is accompanied by his persistent efforts to make his wife miserable when she turns him down, the wrongdoing is less apparent. The husband who repeatedly and roughly kicks the mattress where his wife is trying to sleep, all in an effort to convert her sexual refusal into sexual compliance, does not necessarily seem comparable to a rapist. Even after the husband begins kicking the door when his wife moves to a different bedroom, we may not call it sexual coercion. Indeed, her exhausted and strained "yes," is often taken as proof of her sexual consent. She may not even have to say "yes" to pass as a consenting partner. Just unlocking her door may be enough.[25]

It's not only the appearance of "voluntariness" that makes us dismissive. It also goes unreported and unseen because journalists, scholars, and therapists rarely take an interest. The *banality* of nonviolent sexual coercion, to appropriate Hannah Arendt's term, makes it seem unworthy of attention.

Where Do We Go from Here?

What has been done is one thing, and what can be done is another. People can change, and so can institutions. Sex therapy emerging from work with lesbian partners gives us reason to hope that sex therapy can be operate outside the gender biases that have harmed not only women and their relationships but men too. The assumption that a man has a right to have intercourse with his wife, whether she likes it or not, dehumanizes both her and him. Treating a sexual partner as someone who owes her body to you, not only objectifies her, it isolates him because it stifles the development of his capacity for empathy. Thus, in the spirit of hope for positive change for both women and men, I end with these simple, mostly self-evident suggestions and recommendations:

- In so far as sex therapy's problem is denying women a voice, the remedy is to give women a voice. Let women tell their sexual stories and consider these stories to be as "true" as men's. As Rae Langton put it, "let women into the club of the credible, let women's knowledge count as the knowledge it is."[26]
- The recommendation to "give women a voice" is especially relevant to those who have been deprived of a voice in sexual activity, either as children or adults. When women have been sexually coerced, their power is taken away, and the remedy, again, is to reverse that dynamic in therapy. Give women's power back by asking women who have experienced abuse/coercion, "What would be helpful to you and what would not be helpful? What do you need?"
- Then take in what she says. Hear her.
- Louise Antony offers a suggestion for how this sort of hearing should be done. She says that it makes sense for therapists to adopt "a kind of epistemic affirmative action: to adopt the *working hypothesis* that when a woman, or any member of a stereotyped group, says something anomalous, they should assume that it's *they* who don't understand, not that it's the woman who is nuts."[27]
- Sex therapists should also try to heed Germaine Greer's advice: "No sex rather than bad sex should be an option,"[28] and "bad sex" should never be required either by the partner or therapist.
- In other words, under no circumstances, should a therapist require or encourage or attempt to train anyone to engage in sex they do not want. The harms, and possible harms, from unwanted sex, particularly when they

recur as a routine part of someone's life, can be profound and should discourage a sex therapist from ever advising anyone, in any fashion, to give in to another's sexual demands.
- At the same time, if a woman makes the choice on her own to engage in unpleasurable, even painful sex, to please her partner, preserve her marriage, or for some other reason she finds valid and compelling, the therapist should hear her out. The therapist should be open to discussing the advantages and disadvantages of any sexual decision she is contemplating.
- The therapist should also be open to the idea that a couple, whether in a marriage or any other kind of committed relationship, may find the cost of preserving their relationship too high and that divorce or separation may be the more reasonable option. .
- Both partners should be involved in these discussions. Both should have an opportunity to understand what sex means to them individually and to one another. Partners should discuss what sex means to them as soon as possible because sexual activity, and the need for sexual activity, are often stand-ins for something else. And more often than not, that something else is love. Couples may say they want more sex, but what they're really looking for may be something more akin to emotional connection, a feeling of heightened security and closeness.
- To better develop their understanding of sexual consent and nonviolent coercion, sex therapists need to begin interrogating the complexities of those concepts in their research, in their classrooms, and in their therapy practices. Obviously, it is not enough to define sexual coercion as simply "sex without consent," when consent itself can be coerced in any number of ways.
- When dealing with a sexual discrepancy issue, it does not help to give a psychiatric diagnosis to the one who wants sex less, or, for that matter, to the partner who wants sex more. Giving one of the partners a diagnosis is the same as judging that partner to be wrong and in need of change. Partners need to be treated as equals before they can arrive at an equitable and workable resolution to their sexual issues.
- To increase the likelihood that therapy is being conducted on an even playing field, increasing the likelihood that both partners' sexual consent/free will is respected equally, therapy should include a discussion of the partners' relative socio-economic status. Given the inequality of so many relationships, it should include a conversation about how privilege and power are divided between them.
- To further lessen the possibility of coercion—to lessen the possibility that sex therapy is being used to advance one partner's sexual agenda at the

other's expense—the therapist should give both partners time to explain their motivation for seeking help with their sex lives. What kind of help are they seeking? Why are they seeking help now? *How* do they see this as a problem? What does the problem *mean* to them?[29]
- It is time for sex therapists to put to rest the Freudian myth of the innate, natural, continuously flowing stream-of-sexual-energy and to recognize that many healthy, successful people have little interest in sex.[30] It is time to recognize that, ceteris paribus, a partner who wants more sex is not healthier and more normal and that a partner who wants less sex is not suffering from some kind of deficiency. It is time to recognize that people are sexually different and are entitled to desire as much or as little sex as they want. In the words of Eve Kosofsky Sedgwick, it is time to recognize that,

> sexuality makes up a large share of the self-perceived identity of some people, a small share of others'. . . . Some people spend a lot of time thinking about sex, others little or none. . . . Some people like to have a lot of sex, others little or none.[31]

- Accepting the reality of differential sexual desire suggests that sex therapy programs should incorporate discussion and readings about a type of sexual diversity rarely explored and understood—asexuality. By recognizing asexuality as a valid option, whether it be temporary or permanent, therapists might be in a better position to help women and their partners explore alternatives to the cultural stereotype of the hot and lustful relationship we are all supposed to have to qualify as sexually healthy.
- Finally, while men and women may have different ways of engaging in, and appreciating, sex, it is important for sex therapists to understand that these differences are not the problem. The problem is that men's ways of engaging in, and appreciating, sex have been considered normal, while departures from men's sexuality are prone to diagnosis and treatment as abnormal and suboptimal. They have been taken as the standard for judging women's sexuality. The antidote is to recognize that many women have "a different voice" when it comes to sexual matters, a voice that may, for instance, speak in the idiom of personal connection rather than arousal and orgasm.

The antidote is to acknowledge men's and women's differences and to honor them equally.

Acknowledgments

I am indebted to Abby Gross and Katherine Pratt from Oxford University Press for their extraordinary patience and good will. I am also indebted to Meenakshi Gigi Durham from the University of Iowa and Eileen Gambrill from the University of California–Berkeley for reading the manuscript and offering so many helpful suggestions.

I cannot easily state the nature or extent of my indebtedness to Mary Trachsel, my colleague, friend, and spouse, for her contributions to this text. Her ideas on gender, sexuality, and rhetorical analysis challenged and guided me every step of the way. Thank you, Mary.

A version of Chapter 1 was published as "Freud, Dora, and Compulsory Sexuality" in the *Journal of Humanistic Psychology* (2017): DOI: 10.1177/0022167817739744; a version of Chapter 2 was published as "Sexual Frigidity: The Social Construction of Masculine Privilege and Feminine Pathology" in the *Journal of Gender Studies* 26, no. 5 (September 2017): 583–94; portions of Chapters 3, 8, and 10 were published as "Dilators, Q-Tips, and Extortion: How to Train a Woman for Intercourse in the 'Post-Feminist' Era" in the *Journal of Feminist Family Therapy* 29, no. 4 (October 2017): 189–204.

Notes

Introduction

1. Sims, *Clinical Notes on Women's Surgery*, 326–36.
2. Ibid., 334.
3. Ibid., 335–36.
4. See Dr. Thomas G. Morton's "Removal of the Ovaries as a Cure for Insanity," published in 1893. A year later, in his *Diseases of Women*, Dr. Henry J. Garrigues had this to say about cliteridectomy as a treatment for masturbation: "There is no reason why this little bit of flesh should not be removed, and, as it certainly is the most excitable part of the genitals, it is rational to do so in cases of abnormal excitability irresistibly leading to masturbation, ruining the health of the patient, depriving her of her mental faculties, or driving her to suicide," 292.
5. Sims, *Clinical Notes on Women's Surgery*, 336.
6. Madden, "The Treatment of Vaginismus," 131–32.
7. As recently as 1969, Graber, Barber, and O'Rourke, in their article, "Newlywed Apareunia," advocated surgery for newly married women who experienced painful intercourse.
8. Freud, *Fragment of an Analysis of a Case of Hysteria*, 136.
9. Fenichel, *Psychoanalytic Theory of Neurosis*, 175.
10. Foucault, *Discipline and Punish*, 222.
11. In 2015, the US Food and Drug administration approved a drug, Addyi (flianserin) as a treatment for women's low sexual desire. According to the Addyi website, the primary side-effects associated with this drug are "severe low blood pressure and fainting (loss of consciousness)."
12. In 1992, in her article, "Hypoactive Sexual Desire in Heterosexual Women," Richgels wrote, "A major perceptual error that has limited women sexually is the belief that male experience is human experience," 126. Tiefer said much the same thing in her article, "The Social Construction and Social Effects of Sex Research": "Too often in the sexological model of sexuality the normative standard has been men's experience...," 102.
13. Margaret Jackson introduced the term, "the coital imperative" in 1984, in her article, "Sex Research and the Construction of Sexuality: A Tool of Male Supremacy?"
14. In *Straight*, Hanne Blank argues that the historical record is clear about penis-vagina intercourse: "No other sex act enjoys, or has ever enjoyed, universal approbation. No other source of sexual pleasure is as uniformly accepted, or has ever been," 124.
15. Dworkin, *Intercourse*, 59.
16. Abrams, *Sexuality and Its Disorders*, ix.

17. See MacKinnon, "Rape Redefined," 452. These comments from one of Shere Hite's research subjects reflect this belief: "It was a condition of our marriage as it developed, that if I refused him sexually he was insufferable. I think this is a common degradation of women in marriage. But rape is too strong a word, as force was not involved. I felt prostituted, being used as a whore, with no regard for my desires. I think it is a barbaric tradition, that men cannot be refused by women in marriage, and this led to my finding my husband sexually repugnant." *Shere Hite Reader*, 82.
18. In *The Science/Fiction of Sex*, Annie Potts argues that the experience of orgasm has become the measure of sexual competence, health, and well-being in medical discourse. She adds that "in humanist terms, it also represents a 'peak' sexual experience, a form of self-transcendence or self-actualization." She calls this the "orgasmic imperative," 73–74.
19. In Potts' study of orgasm, "Coming, Coming, Gone," one of the male participants described the sequence of penis-vagina penetration, followed by thrusting, and ending in orgasm as a fundamental socio-structural phenomenon: ". . . in and out, and in and out *speeding* up and reaching *climax*, you know, that's . . . kind of a structure I think that's a very important one in our society, you know, starting slow and getting faster and reaching climax and then that's it. (clicks fingers)," 60.
20. Meana, "Elucidating Women's (Hetero)Sexual Desire," 114.
21. West et al., "Prevalence of Low Sexual Desire and Hypoactive Sexual Desire in a Nationally Representative Sample of US Women."
22. Morrison, *The Bluest Eye*.
23. Hare-Mustin and Marecek, *Making a Difference*, 14.
24. Phillips, Braun, and Gavey, "Defining (Hetero)Sex: How Imperative Is the Coital Imperative?" 237.
25. According to Peggy Kleinplatz, in her article, "History of the Treatment of Female Sexual Dysfunction(s)," "The vast majority of women do not have orgasms as a result of penile thrusting during intercourse," 40.
26. Hite, *The Shere Hite Reader*.
27. Kinsey, *Sexual Behavior in the Human Female*, 133, 142, 282–83, 352, 416–18, 453.
28. See Frost and Donovan, "Low Sexual Desire in Women."
29. Hite, *The Shere Hite Reader*, 23.
30. See Baumeister et al., "Is There a Gender Difference in Strength of Sex Drive?" That review of the literature on gender differences in sexual desire found that "across many different studies and measures, men have been shown to have more frequent and intense sexual desires than women, as reflected in spontaneous thoughts about sex, frequency and varieties of sexual fantasies, desired frequency of intercourse. . . . No contrary findings (indicating stronger sexual motivation among women) were found," 150.
31. Nor is this to say that men don't want intercourse to work for women. They do. As one of Hite's research subjects attests in *The Shere Hite Reader*: "There have been several men who seemed to care whether I was happy, but they wanted to make me happy according to their conception of what ought to do it (thrusting harder or longer

or whatever) and acted as if it was damned impertinent of me to suggest that my responses weren't programmed exactly like those of mythical women in the classics of porn," 63–64.
32. Dworkin, *Intercourse*, 161.
33. See Elliott and Umberson, "The Performance of Desire," and Goffman's *Stigma*.
34. Hochschild, *The Managed Heart*.
35. See Fahs, *Performing Sex*, Muehlenhard and Shippee, "Men's and Women's Reports of Pretending Orgasm," and Wiederman, "Pretending Orgasm during Sexual Intercourse."
36. See Elmerstig et al., "Why Do Young Women Continue to Have Sexual Intercourse Despite Pain?"
37. See Elmerstig et al., "Prioritizing the Partner's Enjoyment," McClelland, "Who Is the 'Self' in Self-Reports of Sexual Satisfaction?," and Nicholson and Burr, "What Is Normal about Women's Hetero(Sexual Desire and Orgasm?"
38. Wolpe, *Psychotherapy by Reciprocal Inhibition*, 152.
39. Blank, in *Straight*, credits Kinsey with elevating the orgasm to the status of international unit for measuring sexual pleasure.
40. According to Masters and Johnson in *The Pleasure Bond*, men are not required to give their female partners an orgasm every time they have intercourse: ". . . our concept of it, basically speaking, holds that if a man maintains control long enough to provide the opportunity for his female partner to achieve satisfaction fifty percent of their coital opportunities, he cannot be considered a premature ejaculator," 33.
41. Kuhn, *The Structure of Scientific Revolutions*.
42. Cooper, "An Innovation in the 'Behavioural' Treatment of a Case of Vaginismus."
43. See Tiefer, "A 'New View' Campaign: A Feminist Critique of Sex Therapy and an Alternative Vision."
44. Brotto and Luria, "Sexual Interest/Arousal Disorder in Women."
45. Asexuality is a relatively new term, and as such, large portions of the general public are unfamiliar with it (see Sarah Young's survey, "Three Quarters of People Cannot Define Asexuality"). It's also a relatively complicated, contested term. For example, in Bogaert's "Asexuality," a groundbreaking study of the demography of asexuality, the phenomenon was defined in narrow, absolute terms as a lifetime absence of sexual attraction "to anyone at all." That led to the oft-cited finding that asexuals represent only one percent of the population. By contrast, in more recent years, many have come to define asexuality in broader, more nuanced terms as a phenomenon that occurs on a spectrum, with the asexual people possibly experiencing a range of romantic and sexual feelings (see Chasin's "Considering Asexuality"). This suggests that asexuality is much more common than we originally imagined. To see examples of this diversity online, readers should google "The Asexual Visibility and Education Network" (AVEN).
46. Foucault, "Nietzsche, Genealogy, History," 148, 150.
47. See Meadmore et al., "Getting Tense about Genealogy."
48. Foucault, *Discipline and Punish*, 30–31.

49. Foucault, "A Conversation with Michel Foucault," 201.
50. A version of this chapter was published as "Freud, Dora, and Compulsory Sexuality," in the *Journal of Humanistic Psychology*.
51. Dr. Haden's comments at the 1867 The British Obstetrical Society Meeting are relevant: "As a body who practice among women, we have constituted ourselves, as it were the guardians of their interests, and in many cases, . . . the custodians of their honour (hear, hear). We are in fact, the stronger, and they are the weaker. They are obliged to believe all that we tell them. They are not in a position to dispute anything we say to them, and we may be said to have them at our mercy," 396.
52. A version of this chapter was published as "Sexual Frigidity: The Social Construction of Masculine Privilege and Feminine Pathology" in the *Journal of Gender Studies*.
53. Wilson, "DSM-III and the Transformation of American Psychiatry."
54. Spitzer, "The Diagnostic Status of Homosexuality in *DSM-III*."
55. American Psychiatric Association, *DSM-III*, 6.
56. Spitzer et al., "Medical and Mental Disorder," 659.
57. American Psychiatric Association, *DSM-IV*, 496–97.
58. American Psychiatric Association, *DSM-5*, 302.72 (F52.22).
59. Kaplan, *Aversion Therapy*, 21.
60. See Baumeister et al., "Is There a Gender Difference in Strength of Sex Drive?"
61. According to Kaplan, *Aversion Therapy*, when a man is married to a sexually withholding woman, his choices are: separate, "or, if he is locked into the relationship by his separation anxieties, develop unhappy, ambivalent compromises," 21.
62. This comment from one of Nicola Gavey's respondents confirms that sometimes women will "consent" to unwanted sex because it's the only way their partner will let them get to sleep: "I mean I just wanted to go to sleep really. . . . So, so after maybe an hour of, um, saying, me saying, 'no,' and him saying, 'Oh come on, come on (pause) um I'd finally think 'Oh my, God, I mean (laugh) for a few, for a few hours of rest I may as—Peace and quiet, I may as well. . . . he kept saying, just, just, let me do this or just let me do that and that will be all. And, and, I mean this could go on for an hour, sort of thing, and, I, I mean, I just wanted to go to sleep really . . . when I had a busy day the next morning." "Technologies and Effects of Heterosexual Coercion," 344. See also Gavey's *Just Sex?* 152. Perhaps because this kind of sexual coercion is rarely discussed, Abby's response to the "Spouse Sulking in the North" seemed to portray it as abnormal and rare: "You have tolerated this for 30 years? What you have described is spousal abuse. Most men do not behave the way your husband does, bullying and coercing their wives into marital relations. Please discuss this with a licensed mental health professional. His behavior is off the charts, and you need more help than I can give you in a letter."
63. Caprio, *The Sexually Inadequate Female*, 43–44.
64. Eichenlaub, *The Marriage Art*, 36.
65. Davis, *The Responsibility of Woman*, 34.
66. Tiefer, "A 'New View' Campaign," 23.
67. Ibid., 23.
68. Ibid., 23.

69. Kleinplatz, "Sex Therapy for Vaginismus," 77.
70. Shaw, "Treatment of Primary Vaginismus," 48.
71. Foucault, *Archaeology of Knowledge*, 32.
72. Fricker, *Epistemic Injustice*, 14.
73. Frye, *The Politics of Reality*, 70.
74. Dworkin, *Intercourse*, 79–80.
75. Brecher, *The Sex Researchers*.
76. Van de Velde, *The Ideal Marriage*, 59.

Chapter 1

1. Foucault, *History of Sexuality*, 151.
2. Ibid., 63.
3. According to Lundberg and Farnham in *Modern Woman*, "Sexuality to Freud included all creative powers, sexual and nonsexual. Creations of art, thought and artisanship Freud regarded as sublimations of sexuality, as sexual drives deflected to another socially approved level. Friendship, comradeship and fellowship as well as parental love were all, to Freud, aspects of fundamental sexuality," 246.
4. Cole, *Sex in Christianity and Psychoanalysis*, 217.
5. Freud, "Recommendations to Physicians Practicing Psychoanalysis," 360.
6. Wortis, *Fragments of a Freudian Analysis*, 845.
7. Marcus, *Freud, Dora: Story, History, Case History*, 85.
8. Moi, "Representation of Patriarchy: Sexuality and Epistemology in Freud's Dora," 191.
9. Katz, *The Invention of Heterosexuality*, 71.
10. Kahane, "Why Dora Now?" 20.
11. See Emens, *Compulsory Sexuality*, also Gupta, "Compulsory Sexuality."
12. See Dotson, "Tracking Epistemic Violence."
13. Malcolm, *Psychoanalysis: The Impossible Profession*.
14. Dora, whose real name is Ida Bauer, was born on November 1, 1882.
15. Freud, *Fragment of an Analysis of a Case of Hysteria*, 126.
16. Ibid., 126.
17. Freud overstated Dora's age by saying that only one year, rather than two, elapsed between Herr K.'s two seduction attempts. Contemporary scholars agree that Dora was actually about 13½ years at the time of Herr K.'s first seduction attempt (see Mahoney, *Freud's Dora*).
18. Freud, *Fragment of an Analysis of a Case of Hysteria*, 43.
19. Ibid., 45.
20. Ibid., 46.
21. Ibid., 53.
22. Ibid., 54.
23. Ibid., 32.
24. Ibid., 53.

25. Ibid., 64.
26. Ibid., 65.
27. Ibid., 68–69.
28. MacMillan, *Freud Evaluated: The Completed Arc*.
29. Freud, *Fragment of an Analysis of a Case of Hysteria*, 71.
30. Ibid., 73.
31. Ibid., 74.
32. Ibid., 74.
33. Ibid., 74–75.
34. Ibid., 75.
35. Ibid., 76.
36. Ibid., 76.
37. Ibid., 81.
38. Ibid., 83.
39. Ibid., 87.
40. Ibid., 87–88.
41. Ibid., 88.
42. Ibid., 82.
43. Ibid., 89.
44. Ibid., 90.
45. Ibid., 90.
46. Ibid., 94.
47. Ibid., 94.
48. Ibid., 94.
49. Ibid., 94.
50. Malcolm, *Psychoanalysis: The Impossible Profession*, 73.
51. Freud, *Fragment of an Analysis of a Case of Hysteria*, 95.
52. Ibid., 95.
53. Ibid., 96.
54. Ibid., 97; emphasis added.
55. Jung, *Memories, Dreams, Reflections*, 147.
56. Ibid., 147.
57. Kazin, "The Freudian Revolution Analyzed," 15.
58. Tatchell, "Freud and the Liberation of Sexual Desire."
59. Bogaert, "Asexuality."
60. Carrigan, "There's More to Life than Sex?"
61. See Chasin, "Theoretical Issues in the Study of Asexuality" and "Reconsidering Asexuality and Its Radical Potential."

Chapter 2

1. Freud, *Three Essays on Sexuality*, 62.
2. Ibid., 62.
3. Bergler, *Counterfeit Sex*, 170.

4. Bergler and Kroger, *Kinsey's Myth of Female Sexuality*, 168.
5. Robinson, *The Power of Sexual Surrender*, 46.
6. Ellis, *Studies in the Psychology of Sex*.
7. To understand why frigidity discourse became so popular with male physicians, it may be helpful to consider that it offered them an opportunity to eroticize the power differential between men and women, particularly the power differential associated with intercourse. As gynecologist Robert H. Fagan wrote in the *Western Journal of Surgery, Obstetrics, & Gynecology*, in an article titled, "Management of the couple with the Problem of Unsuccessful Intercourse" (1958): "Whether it is the touch of her hand, the fragrance of her hair, the fathomless depth of her eyes, the curve of her ankles, the softness of her breasts, or her kisses sweeter than wine, it is all the varying degrees of sex appeal. The summation of this is successful intercourse by which we mean sincere and stimulating love play; intercourse with increasing, joyous crescendo and complete fulfillment in ecstatic, simultaneous climaxes." Ironically, the physician who waxed poetically about the "fathomless depth" of a woman's eyes and "her kisses sweeter than wine," also wrote this in the very same article: "It is incredible and appalling how many times a woman will be well-groomed externally, but not internally. She will carefully shave her underarms and legs too, but her vulva may be a veritable forest of long vulvar hair. Not only this, but many times the vulva will be caked in areas with smegma which often extends under the clitoral folds and causes an unpleasant odor. Moreover, her nipples will be partially covered with sticky discharge from her breasts. Now, of course, this is not true of the majority of women. I think, by and large, our American women are clean and neat, but the opposite occurs so frequently that it exists as a real factor in unsuccessful intercourse," 302–305.
8. Kroger and Freed, "Psychoanalytic Aspects of Frigidity," 526.
9. Gillett, "Normal Frigidity in Women," 29–32.
10. Anonymous review of Oliven's *Sexual Hygiene and Pathology*, 531.
11. Koedt, *The Myth of the Vaginal Orgasm*, 11.
12. Freud, *New Introductory Lectures on Psychoanalysis*, 180.
13. Bergler, "The Problem of Frigidity," 389.
14. Angel, "Contested Psychiatric Ontology and Feminist Critique."
15. Hitschmann and Bergler, *Frigidity in Women*, 20; emphasis added.
16. Bergler, *Divorce Won't Help*, 79–80.
17. Ibid., 79–80.
18. Bergler, "Newer Genetic Investigation on Impotence and Frigidity," 50.
19. Ibid., 50.
20. Ibid., 50.
21. Bergler, *Divorce Won't Help*, 80.
22. Bergler, "The Problem of Frigidity," 382.
23. Ibid., 382.
24. Hitschmann and Bergler, *Frigidity in Women*, 23, 48.
25. Hartogs, "Analyst's Couch," 60. In 1976, a New York court convicted this psychiatrist of sexually abusing a patient on his office couch, a crime for which he was fined $25,000, and which represented the first successful prosecution of this type of sexual abuse (see Roy v. Hartogs, 381 N.Y.S. 2nd 587).

26. Ibid.
27. Ibid.
28. Hitschmann and Bergler, *Frigidity in Women*, 43.
29. Ibid., 38–39.
30. Robinson, *The Power of Sexual Surrender*, 117–22.
31. Bergler and Kroger, *Kinsey's Myth of Female Sexuality*, 87.
32. Quoted in Ehrenreich and English, *For Her Own Good*, 298.
33. Lundberg and Farnham, *Modern Woman*, 108.
34. Chideckel, *Female Sex Perversions*, 272.
35. Robinson, *The Power of Sexual Surrender*, 98.
36. Ibid., 98.
37. Quoted in Stekel, *Frigidity in Woman*, 264.
38. Bonaparte, "Passivity, Masochism, and Femininity," 327.
39. Ibid., 118.
40. Quoted in Stone and Stone, *A Marriage Manual*, 256.
41. Bergler and Kroger, *Kinsey's Myth of Female Sexuality*, 184.
42. Bergler, "The Problem of Frigidity," 389.
43. Ibid., 389.
44. Caprio, *The Sexually Adequate Female*, 145.
45. Ibid., 147.
46. Ibid., 147.
47. Bergler, "The Problem of Frigidity," 380.
48. Hitschmann and Bergler, *Frigidity in Women*, 51.
49. Bergler, "Newer Genetic Investigations on Frigidity and Impotence," 57.
50. Bergler, *Divorce Won't Help*, 70.
51. Ibid., 70.
52. Bergler, *Conflict in Marriage*, 110–11.
53. Ibid., 110–11.
54. Ibid., 110–11.
55. Robinson, *The Power of Sexual Surrender*, 72.
56. Fricker, *Epistemic Injustice*, 162.
57. Hitschmann and Bergler, *Frigidity in Women—Restatement and Renewed Experiences*, 51.
58. Bergler and Kroger, *Kinsey's Myth of Female Sexuality*, 71.
59. Bergler and Kroger, "The Dynamic Significance of Vaginal Lubrication to Frigidity," 713.
60. Kroger and Freed, *Psychosomatic Gynecology*, 295.
61. Bergler, "The Problem of Frigidity," 379.
62. Hitschmann and Bergler, *Frigidity in Women*, 20–21.
63. Ibid.
64. Robinson, *Married Life and Happiness*, 84.
65. Hitschmann and Bergler, *Frigidity in Women*, 50–57.
66. Chideckel, *Female Sex Perversions*, 265.
67. Ibid., 265.

68. Robinson, *The Power of Sexual Surrender*, 43.
69. Ibid., 133.
70. Hitschmann and Bergler, *Frigidity in Women*, 5.
71. Lazarus, "The Treatment of Chronic Frigidity by Systematic Desensitization," 273.
72. Hamilton, "Frigidity in the Female," 1041.
73. Ibid., 1041.
74. Caprio, *The Sexually Adequate Female*, 84, 44.
75. Ibid., 14.
76. Hamilton, "Frigidity in the Female," 1047.
77. Hitschmann and Bergler, *Frigidity in Women*, 5.
78. Bergler, *Divorce Won't Help*, 216.
79. Bergler, "The Problem of Frigidity," 385.
80. Bergler, *Divorce Won't Help*, 217.
81. Dunbar, *Emotions and Bodily Changes*, 534.
82. Bergler, "The Problem of Frigidity," 382.
83. Hamilton, "Frigidity in the Female," 1049.
84. Robinson, *The Power of Sexual Surrender*, 32.
85. Hamilton, "Frigidity in the Females," 1046.
86. Ibid., 1046.
87. Robinson, *The Power of Sexual Surrender*, 135.
88. Ibid., 149.
89. Ibid., 155–56.
90. Ibid., 158.
91. Friedan, *The Feminine Mystique*, 36.

Chapter 3

1. Elliott, "The Use of 'Impotence' and 'Frigidity.'"
2. May, *Homeward Bound*.
3. In 1977, in "The Professionalization of Sex Therapy," LoPicollo wrote, "It was only with the landmark publication of Master's and Johnson's Human Sexual Inadequacy (1970) that the general public became aware of the existence of a new and effective 'sex therapy,'" 513.
4. Quoted in Morrow, *Sex Research and Sex Therapy*, 157.
5. Rosen and Leiblum, in their article, "Assessment and Treatment of Desire Disorders," wrote: "The importance of their contributions cannot be overemphasized, as Masters and Johnson provided a quantum leap forward from the earlier psychodynamic formulations of female 'frigidity.'" 20. See also Bancroft, *Human Sexuality and Its Problems*.
6. Kaplan, *The New Sex Therapy*, 3–4.
7. Masters and Johnson, "Principles of the New Sex Therapy," 548.
8. Ibid., 548.

9. Quoted in LoPicollo, "The Direct Treatment of Sexual Dysfunction," 1227.
10. Beard, *Woman as Force in History*.
11. Millett, in *Sexual Politics*, described Freud as "beyond question the strongest individual counterrevolutionary force in the ideology of sexual politics," 178.
12. Densmore, "Independence from the Sexual Revolution," 103.
13. Kinsey, *Sexual Response in the Human Female*.
14. Irvine, *Disorders of Desire*, 45–46.
15. Masters and Johnson, *Human Sexual Response*, 60.
16. Koedt, "The Myth of the Vaginal Orgasm," 207.
17. Masters in Masters and Johnson, "The Playboy Interview," 168.
18. Johnson in Masters and Johnson, "The Playboy Interview," 169.
19. Morrow, *Sex Research and Sex Therapy*.
20. Masters and Johnson, *Human Sexual Response*, 7, 65, 131.
21. Masters and Johnson, Human Sexual Inadequacy, 219.
22. Masters and Johnson, *Human Sexual Inadequacy*, 219–20.
23. Irvine, *Disorders of Desire*. In *Disorders of Desire*, Janice Irvine argued that Masters and Johnson felt that men were overburdened with an "unconscionable responsibility for sexual interaction," a point she supported with this passage from *Human Sexual Inadequacy*: "The most unfortunate misconception our culture has assigned to sexual functioning is the assumption, by both men and women, that men by divine guidance and infallible instinct are able to discern exactly what a woman wants sexually and when she wants it. Probably this fallacy has interfered with natural sexual interaction as much as any other single factor. The second most frequently encountered sexual fallacy, and therefore a constant deterrent to effective sexual expression, is the assumption, again by both men and women, that sexual expertise is the man's responsibility," 147.
24. Ibid., 117–18.
25. Jackson, "Sex Research and the Construction of Sexuality," 47.
26. Ibid., 173.
27. Ibid., 345.
28. Ibid., 346.
29. Ibid., 346.
30. Dahl, "The Concept of Power," 202–203.
31. Jackson and Scott, "Embodying Orgasm," 106.
32. See Brady's *Fathers Days*. Also see Morber's "What Science Says About Arousal During Rape."
33. Borreli, "Faking Orgasms."
34. E.g., Lydon, *The Politics of Orgasm*, and Hamblin, "The Suppressed Power of Female Sexuality."
35. Masters and Johnson, *Human Sexual Response*, 68, 80.
36. Ibid., 311.
37. Ibid., 315.
38. Masters and Johnson, *Human Sexual Inadequacy*, 255.
39. Ibid., 255.
40. Masters and Johnson, *Human Sexual Response*, 189; emphasis added.

41. Ibid., 128.
42. Ibid., 128.
43. Irvine, *Disorders of Desire*, 65.
44. Masters and Johnson, *Human Sexual Inadequacy*, 328–29.
45. Masters and Johnson, *Human Sexual Response*, 246.
46. See Masters and Johnson, *Human Sexual Inadequacy*, 92–315.
47. Ibid., 131.
48. Ibid., 131.
49. Ibid., 206.
50. Ibid., 207.
51. Ibid., 208.
52. Ibid., 208.
53. Ibid., 92.
54. Ibid., 209.
55. Ibid., 306–307.
56. Ibid., 260; emphasis added.
57. Ibid., 258–59.
58. Ibid., 267.
59. Masters and Johnson, "The Playboy Interview," 148.
60. Ibid., 147.
61. Shere Hite's comments on this issue in the *Shere Hite Reader* are interesting and important: "There is nothing wrong with saying that the movement of the clitoral hood over the clitoris is what is responsible for the orgasm; this is true. What is wrong is to say that thrusting in itself will activate this mechanism in most women. As Alix Shulman has pointedly remarked, Masters and Johnson observe that the clitoris is automatically 'stimulated' in intercourse, since the hood covering the clitoris is pulled over the clitoris with each thrust of the penis in the vagina—much, I suppose, as a penis can be automatically 'stimulated' by a man's underwear when he takes a step.

    "But let's apply this same logic to men. As Dr. Sanford Copley put it, when interviewed on the television show *Woman*, this indirect stimulation of women could be compared to the stimulation that would be produced in a man by the rubbing of the scrotal skin (balls), perhaps pulling it back and forth, and so causing the skin of the upper tip of the penis to move, or quiver, and in this way achieving 'stimulation.' Would it work? Admittedly, this form of stimulation would probably require a good deal more foreplay for the man to have an orgasm! You would have to be patient and 'understand' if it did not lead to orgasm 'every time,'" 57.
62. See Kleinplatz, "History of the Treatment of Female Sexual Dysfunctions(s)."
63. Masters and Johnson, *The Pleasure Bond*. This passage illustrates, perhaps better than any other, Masters and Johnson's belief in the importance of intercourse for a successful heterosexual relationship: "If a man and woman are committed to the enjoyment of their own sexual natures and to each other as sexual persons, intercourse allows them to express their emotions in whatever ways seem desirable and appropriate at the moment, revealing themselves not only to each other—but to themselves. By responding freely to the urgencies of their own bodies as well as to the urgings of their partner, their actions embody their feelings. Liberated from the domination of

reason and discipline, they are able to communicate spontaneous wishes that need no justification," 267.
64. Ibid., 262.
65. Masters and Johnson, "Principles of the New Sex Therapy," 549.
66. Hall, "Not Tonight, Dear," 162.
67. Masters and Johnson, "Principles of the New Sex Therapy," 549.
68. Ibid., 549.
69. Masters and Johnson, *Human Sexual Inadequacy*, 39–47.
70. Ibid., 230–31.
71. Ibid., 264.
72. Kaplan, *The New Sex Therapy*, 209.
73. Masters and Johnson, *Human Sexual Inadequacy*, 31.
74. Ibid., 12.
75. Ibid., 12–13; emphasis in original.
76. See Hunter, *Treatise on Venereal Disease*, as quoted in William Acton's *Practical Treatise on the Diseases of the Urinary and Generative Organs in Both Sexes*. Hunter offered the following example of how he treated a man who lost his "virility" as a result of his overly intense need to perform intercourse successfully with a particular woman: "I told him that he might be cured if he could perfectly rely on his own power of self-denial. When I explained what I meant, he told me that he could depend upon every act of his will, or resolution; I then told him, if he had a perfect confidence in himself in that respect, that he was to go to bed to this woman, but first promise to himself that he would not have any connexion with her for six nights, let his inclinations and powers be what they would, which he engaged to do, and also to let me know the result. About a fortnight after he told that his resolution had produced such a total alteration in the state of his mind that the power soon took place; for instead of going to bed with the fear of inability, he went with fears that he should be possessed with too much desire, too much power, so as to become uneasy to him, which really happened; for he would have been happy to have shortened the time; and when he had once broke the spell, the mind and powers went on together, and his mind never returned to its former state," 181.
77. Masters and Johnson, *Human Sexual Inadequacy*, 13.
78. Ibid., 103.
79. Ibid., 307.
80. For a summary of this literature, see McCormick, *Sexual Salvation*, 180–86.
81. Gill and Walker, "Heterosexuality, Feminism, Contradiction," 455.
82. Hite, *The Hite Report*.

Chapter 4

1. See Willyard, "Men: A Growing Minority?" Also see Carey, "Need Therapy?"
2. Barry, *Female Sexual Slavery*, 172.
3. Goodwach, "Sex Therapy."

4. Richgels, "Hypoactive Sexual Desire in Heterosexual Women."
5. Kaplan, *The New Sex Therapy*, 359.
6. Ibid., 359.
7. Quoted in Irvine, *Disorders of Desire*, 153.
8. Manne, *Down Girl*, 197.
9. Kaplan, *Sexual Aversion*, 128.
10. Ibid., 128.
11. Hochschild, *The Second Shift*, 45.
12. Ibid.
13. Kaplan, *Sexual Aversion*, 130.
14. Ibid., 128.
15. These comments are from one of Elliott and Umberson's research subjects, in "The Performance of Desire," 399.
16. Dworkin, *Intercourse*, 208.
17. See Fahs and Swank, "The Other Third Shift?" To clarify, the regular "third shift" for Hochschild consists of the time women need to balance and reconcile their choices and decisions during their first two shifts. While sex therapists often explain women's lack of sexual interest as a psychological problem, their disinterest can also be understood as a function of sheer exhaustion given all the work they are supposed to do on their first three shifts. In other words, women may simply too tired—too overwhelmed by the responsibilities they are already dealing with—to get interested in their "other third shift." Elliott and Umberson, in their article, "The Performance of Desire," illustrate this phenomenon with the case of Maria who "was more concerned about the bills, the kids, daily routines, things that needed to get done. Dishes, even dishes or laundry, that kind of stuff, was already a priority first before any leisure time at all or sex, or whatever," 14.
18. See Hare-Mustin, "Discourses in the Mirrored Room."
19. Kaplan, *The New Sex Therapy*, 229.
20. Ibid., 371.
21. Ibid., 371–72.
22. Stephenson and Meston, "Consequences of Impaired Female Sexual Functioning."
23. Ibid., 372.
24. Ibid., 372.
25. Ibid., 372.
26. Ibid., 372.
27. Sanchez et al., "Sexual Submissiveness in Women."
28. Kaplan, *The New Sex Therapy*, 371.
29. Ibid., 373.
30. Kaplan, *The Sexual Desire Disorders*, 4.
31. Kaplan, *Disorders of Sexual Desire*, 38.
32. Kaplan, *The New Sex Therapy*, 230.
33. Ibid., 230.
34. *McCormick, Sexual Salvation*. McCormick commented, "Sex therapists are all too quick to assume that women should be constantly ready for sex if their partner is attractive, loving, and appropriate (whatever that means)," 190.

35. Ibid., 230–31.
36. Ibid., 231.
37. Ibid., 231.
38. Ibid., 231–32.
39. Kaplan, *The Sexual Desire Disorders*, 86–89.
40. Ibid., 87.
41. Hayles, "Anger in Different Voices."
42. Kaplan, *The Sexual Desire Disorders*, 86.
43. Ibid., 88.
44. Ibid., 86.
45. See Tuana, "The Speculum of Ignorance," 13.
46. See Hare-Mustin, "Discourses in the Mirrored Room."

Chapter 5

1. Hartman and Fithian, *Treatment of Sexual Dysfunction*, 121–23.
2. Ibid., 123.
3. As William Hartman put it in "Sexual Myths," "Sex is something you do, not something you talk about," 19.
4. In what way is the expression of power through heterosexual intercourse "very, very fulfilling" to a man. Andrea Dworkin's answer in *Intercourse* is "ownership." A husband can own his wife's property, he can claim the benefits of her work, he can claim the benefits of everything she does, but penetrating her vagina with his penis, according to Dworkin, "getting inside and owning [her] insides is possession deeper, more intimate, than any other kind of ownership. Intimate, raw, total, the experience of sexual possession for women is real and literal, without and magical or mystical dimension to it: getting fucked and being owned are inseparably the same; together, being one and the same, they are sex for women under male dominance as a social system," 83.
5. Irvine, *Disorders of Desire*, 85.
6. Hartman and Fithian, *Treatment of Sexual Dysfunction*, 89.
7. Ibid., 81.
8. Ibid., 81.
9. Ibid., 94–95.
10. Ibid. For example, Hartman and Fithian had women rapidly contract and relax their pubococcygeus muscle twenty-five to fifty times a day, an activity that supposedly approximates women's involuntary contractions during orgasm. They also had their women patients take "a deep breath, pulling up from the vagina at the same time tightening up the genital muscles then relaxing the whole pelvic region as air is exhaled." Women had to do ten of these per day. Other exercises included asking women to bear down "s though they were going to expel something from their vagina," as though simulating childbirth, "then tightening up the muscle after ceasing to bear down," 87.
11. Ibid., 89.

12. Irvine, *Disorders of Desire*, 88.
13. Hartman and Fithian, "Non-Orgasmic Women Study."
14. Marilyn Fithian's obituary by Elaine Woo, appeared in the *Los Angeles Times* on September 19, 2008, and placed her and Hartman on a par with Kinsey and Masters and Johnson: "She and Hartman, who died in 1997, were sometimes described as the Masters and Johnson of the West Coast whose contributions to their field were considered as important as those of Kinsey and the team of Masters and Johnson: 'They helped legitimize and destigmatize sex research,' wrote Eli Coleman, a past president of the Society for the Scientific Study of Sexuality and the Director of the human sexuality program at the University of Minnesota. He described their book as one of the most important in the field during the 1970s, along with Masters and Johnson's landmark work Human Sexual Response."
15. Ibid.
16. Lazarus, "The Treatment of Chronic Frigidity by Systematic Desensitization."
17. Ibid., 275.
18. Ibid., 275.
19. Ibid., 275.
20. Ibid., 275.
21. Foucault, *Discipline and Punish*, 94.
22. De Shazer, "Some Conceptual Distinctions Are More Useful Than Others."
23. Shrifren et al., "Sexual Problems and Distress in United States Women."
24. Wolpe, "The Treatment of Inhibited Sexual Responses," 52; emphasis added.
25. It's interesting that in "The Treatment of Inhibited Sexual Responses," Wolpe does not observe that people, in general, occasionally fail to develop a normal sexual response system. He only mentions women.
26. Wolpe, *The Practice of Behavior Therapy*, 88.
27. Lazarus, "The Treatment of Chronic Frigidity by Systematic Desensitization," 276.
28. Ibid., 276.
29. Wolpe, *Psychotherapy by Reciprocal Inhibition*, 132.
30. Ibid., 132.
31. Ibid., 131; emphasis in original.
32. Wolpe, *The Practice of Behavior Therapy*, 85.
33. Ibid., 86–87.
34. Zussman et al., "Treatment of a Case of Vaginal Constriction Preventing Coitus."
35. Ibid., 105.
36. In the following passage from *Treatment of Sexual Dysfunction*, Hartman and Fithian caution women against ever saying "no" to their male partner's sexual advances by offering the following anecdote: "Several years ago while observing a research couple in coitus, the female in the midst of coital activities said to her partner very loudly 'stop.' Needless to say, the entire lovemaking activities halted. All the enjoyable feelings and the degree of arousal which had been present went 'down the drain,' and then in a somewhat embarrassing and uncomfortable situation, both partners attempted to continue their lovemaking activities—never fully recovering the momentum well underway at 'stop.'"

As Hartman and Fithian continue, their warning against use of the "no" word in sexual situations becomes explicit: "In the video tapes of sexual functioning the couples who seem to function best are the ones who are always saying yes to the lovemaking activities in which they are involved. The implicit suggestion here is that couples encourage their partners, and engage in those activities which they do enjoy, reaffirming by saying yes that they are enjoying the activity. . . . A negative response often seriously inhibits further lovemaking efforts and, therefore, should be avoided wherever possible," 186.
37. Brady, "Brevital-Relaxation Treatment of Frigidity," 77.
38. Wijma and Wijma, "A Cognitive Behavioural Treatment Model of Vaginismus," 150.
39. Cooper, "An Innovation in the 'Behavioural Treatment of a Case of Nonconsummation Due to Vaginismus."
40. Ibid., 721.
41. Ibid., 721.
42. Ibid., 721.
43. Ibid., 721.
44. Reissing et al., "Does Vaginismus Exist? A Critical Review of the Literature," 265; emphasis added.
45. Ibid., 722; emphasis added.
46. I connected the treatment described in this paper to rape in my paper, "Dilators, Q-tips, and Extortion: How to Train a Woman for Intercourse in the 'Post-Feminist' Era." The total number of citations (38) for this study reflects what I found the last time I checked Google Scholar (September 28, 2018).
47. Ibid., 722.

Chapter 6

1. Wilson, "DSM-III and the Transformation of American Psychiatry."
2. Spitzer, "The Diagnostic Status of Homosexuality in the *DSM-III*."
3. Spitzer et al., "Medical and Mental Disorder."
4. American Psychiatric Association, *DSM-III*, 278; emphasis added.
5. See Bayer, *Homosexuality and American Psychiatry*, 127.
6. Spitzer et al., *DSM-III Case Book*, 96–97.
7. The case of Mr. and Ms. B., appears, in some ways, strikingly similar to a case study, "Luz," published in Ventura, *Casebook for DSM-5*. Like the Mr. and Ms. B. case, the description of Luz's motivation for seeking sex therapy is presented in the vaguest possible terms: "She came to counseling owing to sexual problems in her marriage and wants to be 'happy with her husband,'" 123.
8. Ibid. This sentence is also very similar to one from the "Luz" case study: "David [the husband] has been patient for the past 10 years but is increasingly becoming frustrated with the lack of her willingness to engage in physical intimacy," 124.
9. Donahey, "Problems with Orgasm," 182.

10. See Nicholson and Burr, "What Is 'Normal' about Women's (Hetero)Sexual Desire and Orgasm?"
11. Ibid., 63.
12. Donahey, "Problems with Orgasm," 189.
13. Kleinplatz, "Sex Therapy and Vaginismus," 67.
14. Lieblum, "Preface," xii.
15. Basson, "Sexual Desire/Arousal Disorders in Women," 38.
16. Ibid., 39.
17. Ibid., 39.
18. West in her article, "The Harms of Consensual Sex," writes, "Let us assume what many women who are or have been heterosexually active surely know to be true from their own experience, and that is some women occasionally, and many women quite frequently, consent to sex even when they do not desire the sex itself, and accordingly have a good deal of sex that, although consensual, is in no way pleasurable," 371.
19. See Fahs et al., "I Just Go with It," and Herbenick et al., "Sexual Desire Discrepancy."
20. In "The Performance of Desire," Elliott and Umberson refer to wives who view sexual interaction as a payment their spouse has earned in exchange for the performance of household chores, 14.
21. Basile, "Prevalence of Wife Rape and Other Intimate Partner Sexual Coercion in a Nationally Representative Sample of Women," 516.
22. Ibid., 516.
23. Ibid. The following list represents the conditions that Basile used to measure the prevalence of sexual coercion:

    1 when you thought he expected sex from you in return for certain actions, such as spending money on you for a gift or taking you out for a nice dinner.
    2 because you thought it was your duty to have sex with him when he wants to have sex.
    3 after a romantic situation, such as a back rub or intimate kissing.
    4 after he begged and pleaded with you to have sex.
    5 after he said things to bully/humiliate you into having sex.
    6 after he threatened to hurt you if you did not have sex.
    7 after he used physical force on you in order to have sex, 516.

24. Quoted in Rich, *Of Woman Born*, 41.
25. Rich, *Of Woman Born*, 41.
26. Drye, "The Startling Truth about Sexual Coercion."
27. West, "The Harms of Consensual Sex," 372.
28. Gavey et al., "Interruptus Coitus," 55.
29. Lief, "Integrative Therapy in a Woman with Secondary Low Sex Desire," 110, 129.
30. Rosen and Leiblum, "Preface," x.
31. Ibid., 114.
32. Ibid., 114.
33. Ibid., 115.
34. Kuhn, *The Structure of Scientific Revolutions*, 5.
35. Lief, "Integrative Therapy in a Woman with Secondary Low Sex Desire," 125.

36. Ibid., 125.
37. Ibid., 128.
38. LoPicollo, "Master Series."
39. Bass and Davis, *The Courage to Heal*, 346.
40. Breuer and Freud, *Studies in Hysteria*.
41. See Garfinkel, "Conditions of Successful Degradation Ceremonies."

Chapter 7

1. Gehring, "Couple Therapy for Low Desire," 28.
2. Ibid., 28.
3. Ibid., 28–29.
4. Ibid., 29.
5. Maurice, "Sexual Desire Disorders in Men."
6. Ibid., 202.
7. Ibid., 202.
8. Fraser and Solovey, "A Catalytic Approach to Brief Sex Therapy," 190.
9. Ibid., 190.
10. Ibid., 203.
11. Ibid., 204.
12. Ibid., 205.
13. Ibid., 205.
14. Hall, "Male Hypoactive Sexual Desire Disorder," 67.
15. Fraser and Solovey, "A Catalytic Approach to Brief Sex Therapy," 205.
16. Ibid., 190.
17. Ibid., 190.
18. See MacKinnon, *Sexual Harassment of Working Women*.
19. Fraser and Solovey, "A Catalytic Approach to Brief Sex Therapy," 191.
20. Ibid., 191.
21. Ibid., 207.
22. Ibid., 206.
23. Ibid., 208.
24. Ibid., 209.
25. Ibid., 209.
26. Rich, *Of Woman Born*, 41.
27. Fraser and Solovey, "A Catalytic Approach to Brief Sex Therapy," 190.
28. See Alinsky et al., "Power and Perspectives Not Taken."
29. Du Bois, *The Souls of Black Folk*, 2.
30. Harman et al., "Relationship Enhancement Therapy," 123.
31. Ibid., 124.
32. See Hendrickx et al., "Prevalence Rates of Sex and Difficulties and Associated Distress in Heterosexual Women and Men." Also see Shifren et al., "Sexual Problems and Distress in United States Women."

33. Rosen et al., "Epidemiology."
34. Harman et al., "Relationship Enhancement Therapy," 125.
35. Renshaw, "Sexless Marriages and Sex Therapy," 180.
36. Ibid., 183.
37. Ibid., 183.
38. Ibid., 183.
39. Ibid., 183.
40. Meana and Steiner, "Hidden Disorder/Hidden Desire," 56.
41. Frost and Donovan, "Low Sexual Desire in Women," 344.
42. Elliott and Umberson, "The Performance of Desire," 399–400.
43. The idea that a woman should adapt to a man's sexual needs is not only consistent with sex role stereotypes, it's consistent with women's sexual expectations. According to a recent study of male and female undergraduates by Sanchez et al., "Sexual Submissiveness in Women," women internalize the stereotype of the submissive woman and dominant man at an unconscious level. They also tend to associate sex with submission and are thus more likely to adapt a submissive role in sex.

Chapter 8

1. American Psychiatric Association, *DSM-IV-TR Casebook*, 229.
2. This is how Wiley, the publisher, described the book in its advertising.
3. Carpenter et al., "Treating Women's Orgasmic Difficulties," 65.
4. Ibid., 65.
5. Ibid., 65.
6. Ibid., 65–66.
7. Ibid., 66.
8. Ibid., 65.
9. Weeks et al., "Preface," xxiv.
10. Wylie et al., "Inhibited Arousal in Women," 159.
11. Meana et al. "Treating Genital Pain Associated with Intercourse," 111.
12. Ibid., 111.
13. Ibid., 111.
14. Leiblum et al., "The Treatment of Vaginismus," 123.
15. Ibid., 123.
16. Ibid., 125.
17. Ibid., 125.
18. Ibid., 126.
19. Ibid., 125.
20. Ibid., 125.
21. Ibid., 126.
22. Ibid., 126.
23. Ibid., 127.
24. Dworkin, *Intercourse*, 154.

25. Chakrabarti and Sinha, "Marriage Consummated after 22 Years," 302.
26. Ibid., 302.
27. Ibid., 302.
28. Shaw, "Treatment of Primary Vaginismus," 51.
29. Gabbard, "Foreword," ix.
30. Janata and Kingsberg, "Sexual Aversion Disorder."
31. Ibid., 116.
32. Ibid., 117.
33. Ibid., 117.
34. Ibid., 117.
35. Ibid., 117.
36. Ibid., 118.
37. Elliott and Umberson, "The Performance of Desire," 402–403.
38. Fish et al., "Treating Inhibited Sexual Desire."
39. Ibid., 7.
40. Ibid., 8.
41. Ibid., 10.
42. Ibid., 11.
43. Orwell, *1984*, 175.
44. This passage from Robin West, "Equality Theory, Marital Rape," helps clarify the incredible damage that results from rape and other forms of sexual coercion when they occur and recur in marriage and other long-term relationships: "Eventually, her desires are no longer a product of what she enjoys or what she has learned to enjoy. What the victim of routinized rape within marriage does, sexually, is a product not of what the victim wills but of what her attacker demands. As an immediate consequence, her will becomes a function not of her desires but of his desires. Eventually her desires become a function not of her pleasures, but of his pleasures; she wants literally to please him rather than please herself because to please herself is too dangerous. The victim of marital rape gains survival, but she sacrifices self-sovereignty," 42.

Chapter 9

1. Hall, "Sex Therapy with Lesbian Couples," 147–48.
2. Alonzo, "Working with Same-Sex Couples."
3. Ibid., 381.
4. Lev and Nichols, "Sex Therapy with Lesbian and Gay Couples," 220.
5. Grayer, "Emotionally Focused Therapy for Couples."
6. Ibid., 491.
7. Nichols and Shernoff, "Therapy with Sexual Minorities," 395.
8. Ibid., 396–97.
9. Iasenza, "Multicontextual Sex Therapy with Lesbian Couples," 21.

10. Ibid., 21–22.
11. Ibid., 22.
12. Ibid., 23.

Chapter 10

1. See Foucault, *Power/Knowledge*, 119.
2. Pietsch, "Strategic Treatment of Female Hypoactive Desire," 38.
3. Foucault, *Discipline and Punish*, 304.
4. Ibid., 38.
5. Ibid., 39.
6. Jernigan, "Compassionate Authenticity," 57.
7. Ibid., 57.
8. Ibid., 57–58.
9. Ibid., 58.
10. Ibid., 63.
11. Ibid., 65.
12. Brotto and Luia, "Sexual Interest/Arousal Disorder in Women," 35.
13. Ibid., 35–36.
14. Ibid., 36.
15. Ibid., 36.
16. Ibid., 36–37.
17. Miller et al., "Getting 'in the Mood,'" 92.
18. Ibid., 93.
19. Girard and Wooley, "Using Emotionally Focused Therapy," 723.
20. See Tiefer, "Feminist Critique of Sex Therapy."
21. Ibid. Also see Tiefer "A 'New View' Campaign."
22. Girard and Wooley, "Using Emotionally Focused Therapy," 729.
23. Ibid., 729.
24. Ibid., 729.
25. Ibid., 731.
26. Ibid., 730.
27. Ibid., 731.
28. Ibid., 731.
29. Masters and Johnson, *Human Sexual Inadequacy*, 76.
30. American Psychiatric Association, *Diagnostic and Statistical Manual*.
31. Meanna, "Elucidating Women's (Hetero)Sexual Desire," 18.
32. Graham, "Sexual Dysfunction."
33. Ibid., 232.
34. Ibid., 232.
35. Hare-Mustin, "Sex, Lies, and Headaches."
36. Ibid., 51.

Conclusion

1. See McCormick, *Sexual Salvation*, 190.
2. According to Rosemary Basson, in her article, "Using a Different Model for Female Sexual Response to Address Women's Problematic Low Sexual Desire," "When a relatively large percentage of a sample perceives itself to be abnormal, the validity of the standard of normality may well be questioned. Some 30-50% of women report low sexual desire and we might ask to whom are they comparing themselves," 395.
3. American Psychiatric Association, *DSM-5*, 302.72 (F52.22).
4. Spitzer, "The Diagnostic Status of Homosexuality in the *DSM-III*," 214.
5. Krasnow and Maglio, "Female Sexual Desire," 1.
6. See Bancroft, *Human Sexuality and Its Problems*, and Shifren et al., "Sexual Problems and Distress in United States Women."
7. See Black et al., *DSM-5 Guidebook*, 280.
8. McCormick, *Sexual Salvation*, 192.
9. Pertot, *Perfectly Normal*.
10. Jenkins and Johnston, "Unethical Treatment of Gay and Lesbian People with Conversion Therapy," 561.
11. MacKinnon, *Feminism Unmodified*, 58.
12. Goffman, *Stigma*, 74.
13. Chasin, "Reconsidering Asexuality and Its Radical Potential," 416.
14. Torres and Yllo, "Implications for Policy, Practice, and Future Research," 199. See also Johnson's "A Listening Guide Analysis of Women's Experiences of Unacknowledged Rape," which claims that women's most common way of describing unacknowledged rape is through a voice of uncertainty, and that voice has four central variations: self-blame, normalizing, dismissal, and avoidance.
15. Foucault, *Discipline and Punish*, 170.
16. See Frye, *The Politics of Reality*, 4.
17. Ibid., 9.
18. Dworkin, *Intercourse*, 159.
19. See Torres, "Reconciling Cultural Difference in the Study of Marital Rape."
20. See Impett and Peplau, "Why Some Women Consent to Unwanted Sex with a Dating Partner"; Peterson and Muehlenhard, "Conceptualizing the 'Wantedness' of Women's Consensual and Nonconsensual Sexual Experiences"; Elmerstig et al. "Why Do Young Women Continue to Have Intercourse Despite Pain?"; Gavey *Just Sex?*; and Koss et al., "The Scope of Rape."
21. See Elliott and Umberson, "The Performance of Desire," and Basile, "Prevalence of Wife Rape and Other Intimate Partner Sexual Coercion in a Nationally Representative Sample of Women."
22. MacKinnon, *Sexual Harassment of Working Women*.
23. Johnstone, "A Listening Guide Analysis of Women's Experiences of Unacknowledged Rape," 281.
24. See Koss' "Hidden, Unacknowledged, Acquaintance and Date Rape" and Gavey's *Can a Woman Be Raped and Not Know It?* Both argue that instead of dichotomizing

sexual coercion as rape/not rape, we should begin to think of sexual coercion as a continuum, with rape as an endpoint.
25. To cite Catharine MacKinnon, "Rape Redefined," once more, "In the life of inequality, much routine and sad resignation or worse passes for 'voluntariness' in the sexual setting," 440.
26. Langton, ""Feminism in Epistemology," 134.
27. See Antony, "Sisters, Please, I'd Rather Do It Myself," 89, and Gupta, "What Does Asexuality Teach Us about Sexual Disinterest?"
28. Greer, "A Woman's Duty Is Not Only to Have the Sex She Doesn't Want, But to Enjoy It."
29. A technique that therapists might consider using to help patients explain their motivation for seeking help with their sex lives is solution therapy's "miracle question." That technique involves asking both partners to imagine that one night, while they were sleeping, there was a miracle, and the problem that brought them to therapy was solved. They are then asked, How would they know that the miracle occurred? What would be different? How would their partner know that the miracle occurred without directly explaining it to them? See De Shazer et al., *More Than Miracles*.
30. Sedgwick, *Epistemology of the Closet*, 25.
31. Ibid.

Bibliography

Abrams, Mike. *Sexuality and Its Disorders: Development, Cases, and Treatment*. Los Angeles, CA: SAGE, 2017.

Acton, William. *Practical Treatise on the Diseases of the Urinary and Generative Organs in Both Sexes*. Philadelphia: J. B. Lippincott, 1858.

Alonzo, Daniel J. "Working with Same-Sex Couples." In *Handbook of Couple's Therapy*, edited by Michelle Harway, 370–85. Hoboken, NJ: Wiley, 2005.

American Psychiatric Association. *Diagnostic and Statistical Manual of Mental Disorders*. Washington, DC: American Psychiatric Press, 1952.

American Psychiatric Association. *Diagnostic and Statistical Manual of Mental Disorders*, 3rd ed. Washington, DC: American Psychiatric Press, 1980.

American Psychiatric Association. *Diagnostic and Statistical Manual of Mental Disorders*, 4th ed. Washington, DC: American Psychiatric Press, 1993.

American Psychiatric Association. *Diagnostic and Statistical Manual of Mental Disorders*, 5th ed. Washington, DC: American Psychiatric Press, 2013.

Angel, Katherine. "Contested Psychiatric Ontology and Feminist Critique: 'Female Sexual Dysfunction' and the Diagnostic and Statistical Manual." *History and the Human Sciences*, 25, no. 4 (October 2012): 2–24.

Anonymous Review of John F. Oliven's *Sexual Hygiene and Pathology: A Manual for the Physician*. *Journal of the American Medical Association*, 159, no. 5 (October 1955): 530–31.

Antony, Louise. "Sisters, Please, I'd Rather Do It Myself: A Defense of Individualism in Feminist Epistemology." *Philosophical Topics*, 23, no. 2 (October 1995): 59–94.

Bancroft, John. *Human Sexuality and Its Problems*. London: Elsevier, 2009.

Barry, Kathleen. *Female Sexual Slavery*. New York: New York University Press, 1984.

Basile, Kathleen C. "Prevalence of Wife Rape and Other Intimate Partner Sexual Coercion in a Nationally Representative Sample of Women." *Violence and Victims*, 17, no. 2 (October 2002): 511–24.

Bass, Ellen, and Laura Davis. *The Courage to Heal: A Guide for Women Survivors of Child Sexual Abuse*. New York: Harper Perennial, 1992.

Basson, Rosemary. "Using a Different Model for Female Sexual Response to Address Women's Problematic Low Sexual Desire." *Journal of Sex and Marital Therapy*, 27, no. 5 (October 2001): 395–403.

Basson, Rosemary. "Sexual Desire/Arousal Disorders in Women." In *Principles and Practice of Sex Therapy*, 4th ed., edited by Sandra R. Leiblum, 25–53. New York: Guilford, 2006.

Baumeister, Roy F., Kathleen R. Catanese, and Kathleen D. Vohs. "Is There a Gender Difference in Strength of Sex Drive? Theoretical Views, Conceptual Distinctions, and a Review of Relevant Literature." *Personality and Social Psychology Review*, 5, no. 3 (August 2001): 242–73.

Bayer, Ronald. *Homosexuality and American Psychiatry: The Politics of Diagnosis*. New York: Basic Books, 1981.

Beard, Mary, R. *Woman as Force in History*. New York: Persea Books, 1946.

Becker Howard. *Outsiders*. New York: Free Press, 1963.
Bergler, Edmund. "The Problem of Frigidity." *Psychiatric Quarterly*, 18, no. 3 (September 1944): 374–90.
Bergler, Edmund. "Newer Genetic Investigations on Impotence and Frigidity." *Menninger Clinic Bulletin*, 11, no. 2 (March 1947): 50.
Bergler, Edmund. *Divorce Won't Help*. New York: Liveright, 1948.
Bergler, Edmund. *Conflict in Marriage*. New York: International Universities Press, 1949.
Bergler, Edmund. *Counterfeit Sex: Homosexuality, Impotence, Frigidity*. New York: Grune & Stratton, 1949.
Bergler, Edmund, and William S. Kroger. "The Dynamic Significance of Vaginal Lubrication to Frigidity." *Western Journal of Surgery, Obstetrics, & Gynecology*, 61, no. 12 (December 1953): 711.
Bergler, Edmund, and William S. Kroger. *Kinsey's Myth of Female Sexuality*. New York: Grune & Stratton, 1954.
Binik, Yitzchak, M., and Marta Meanna. "The Future of Sex Therapy: Specialization or Marginalization?" *Archives of Sexual Behavior*, 38, no. 6 (December 2009): 1016–27.
Black, Donald, W., and Jon E. Grant. *DSM-5 Guidebook: The Essential Companion to the Diagnostic and Statistical Manual of Mental Disorders*, 5th ed. Washington, DC: American Psychiatric Publishing, 2014.
Blank, Hanne. *Straight: The Surprisingly Short History of Heterosexuality*. Boston, MA: Beacon Press, 2012.
Bogaert, Anthony, F. "Asexuality: Prevalence and Associated Factors in a National Probability Sample." *Journal of Sex Research*, 41, no. 3 (August 2004): 279–87.
Bonaparte, Marie. "Passivity, Masochism, and Femininity." *International Journal of Psychoanalysis*, 16 (1935): 325–33.
Borreli, Lizette. "Faking Orgasms: Women May Exaggerate Sexual Pleasure to End Unwanted, Forced Encounters," July 11, 2016: www.medicaldaily.com/faking-orgasms-women-sexual-pleasure-forced-sex-391606.
Brady, John Paul. "Brevital-Relaxation Treatment of Frigidity." *Behavior Research and Therapy*, 4, nos. 1–2 (January 1966): 71–77.
Brady, Katherine. *Fathers Days A True Story of Incest*. New York: Seaview Books, 1979.
Brecher, Edward M. *The Sex Researchers*. London: Andre Deutch, 1970.
Breuer, Joseph, and Sigmund Freud. *Studies on Hysteria*, translated by James Strachey. New York: Basic Books, 1891/2000.
Brotto, Lori, and Mijal Luria. "Sexual Interest/Arousal Disorder in Women." In *Principles and Practice of Sex Therapy*, 5th ed., edited by Yitzchak M. Binik and Kathryn S. K. Hall, 17–41. New York: Guilford Press, 2014.
Caprio, Frank S. *The Sexually Adequate Female*. New York: Citadel Press, 1953.
Carey, Benedict. "Need Therapy? A Good Man Is Hard to Find." *New York Times*, May 21, 2011: http://www.nytimes.com/2011/05/22/health/22therapists.html? r=1&hp.
Carpenter, Kristen M., Kristin Williams, and Brett Worly. "Treating Women's Orgasmic Difficulties." In *The Wiley Handbook of Sex Therapy*, edited by Zoe D. Peterson, 57–71. Malden, MA: Wiley, 2017.
Carrigan, Mark. "There's More to Life than Sex? Differences and Commonality within the Asexual Community." *Sexualities*, 14, no. 4 (August 2011): 462–78.
Caruth, Cathy. *Trauma: Explorations in Memory*. Baltimore: Johns Hopkins University Press, 1995.

Chakrabarti, Nandini, and V. K. Sinha. "Marriage Consummated after 22 Years: A Case Report." *Journal of Sex and Marital Therapy*, 28, no. 4 (July 2002): 301–304.

Chasin, C. J. DeLuzio. "Theoretical Issues in the Study of Asexuality." *Archives of Sexual Behavior*, 40, no. 4 (August 2011): 713–23.

Chasin, C. J. DeLuzio. "Reconsidering Asexuality and Its Radical Potential." *Feminist Studies*, 39, no. 2 (January 2013): 405–26.

Chasin, C. J. DeLuzio. "Considering Asexuality as a Sexual Orientation and Implications for Acquired Female Sexual Arousal/Interest Disorder." *Archives of Sexual Behavior*, 46, no. 3 (2017): 631–35.

Chideckel, Maurice. *Female Sex Perversion: The Sexually Aberrated Woman as She Is*. New York: Eugenics, 1935.

Clark, LeMon. *The Enjoyment of Love in Marriage*. New York: New American Library, 1969.

Coetzee, J. M. *Disgrace*. London: Vintage, 1999.

Cole, William Graham. *Sex in Christianity and Psychoanalysis*. New York: Oxford University Press, 1955.

Comer, Ronald J. *Abnormal Psychology*, 5th ed. New York: Worth, 2004.

Cooper, Alan. J. "An Innovation in the 'Behavioural' Treatment of a Case of Nonconsummation Due to Vaginismus." *British Journal of Psychiatry*, 115, no. 523 (June 1969): 721–22.

Dahl, Robert A. "The Concept of Power." *Behavioral Science*, 2, no. 3 (July 1957): 201–15.

Davis, Maxine. *The Sexual Responsibility of Woman*. New York: Dial Press, 1956.

Dennerstein, Lorraine, Jeanne L Alexander, and Allesandra Graziottin. "Sexual Desire Disorders in Women." In *Standard Practice in Sexual Medicine*, edited by Harmut Porst and Jacques Buvat, 315–19. Malden, MA: Blackwell, 2006.

Densmore, Dana. "Independence from the Sexual Revolution." In *Radical Feminism*, edited by Anne Koedt, Ellen Levine, and Anita Rapone, 107–18. New York: Quadrangle Books, 1973.

De Shazer, Steve. "Some Conceptual Distinctions Are More Useful than Others." *Family Process*, 21, no. 1 (March 1982): 71–84.

De Shazer, S., Yvonne Dolan, Harry Korman, Terry Trepper, Eric McCollum, and Insoo Kim Berg. *More than Miracles: The State of Art of Solution-Focused Brief Therapy*. New York: Haworth Press, 2007.

Donahey, Karen M. "Female Orgasmic Disorder." In *Handbook of Clinical Sexuality for Mental Health Professionals*, 2nd ed., edited by Stephen B. Levine, 181–192. New York: Routledge, 2010.

Dotson, Kristie. "Tracking Epistemic Violence, Tracking Practices of Silencing." *Hypatia*, 26, no. 2 (May 2011): 236–57.

Drye, Ashley T. "The Startling Truth about Sexual Coercion," January 4, 2017. Retrieved from: https://goodmenproject.com/sex-relationships/the-startling-truth-about-sexual-coercion-babb/

Du Bois, W. E. B. *The Souls of Black Folk*. New York: Routledge, 1903/2016.

Dunbar, Helen Flanders. *Emotions and Bodily Changes*. New York: Arno Press, 1954.

Dworkin, Andrea. *Intercourse*. New York: Basic Books, 2006.

Eichenlaub, John E. *The Marriage Art*. London: Mayflower-Dell, 1961.

Elliott, Mark L. "The Use of 'Impotence' and 'Frigidity': Why Has 'Impotence' Survived?" *Journal of Sex & Marital Therapy*, 11, no. 1 (March 1985): 51–56.

Elliott, Sinikka, and Debra Umberson. "The Performance of Desire: Gender and the Sexual Negotiation of Long-term Marriages." *Journal of Marriage and the Family*, 70, no. 2 (May 2008): 391–406.

Ellis, Havelock. *Studies in the Psychology of Sex*. New York: Random House, 1936.

Elmerstig, Eva, Barbro Wijma, and Carino Bertero. "Why Do Young Women Continue to Have Sexual Intercourse Despite Pain?" *Journal of Adolescent Health*, 43, no. 4 (October 2008): 357–63.

Elmerstig, Eva, Barbro Wijma, and Katarina Swahnberg. "Prioritizing the Partner's Enjoyment: A Population-based Study on Young Swedish Women with Experience of Pain during Vaginal Intercourse." *Journal of Psychosomatic Obstetrics & Gynecology*, 34, no. 2 (December 2013): 82–89.

Emens, Elizabeth F. "Compulsory Sexuality." *Stanford Law Review*, 66 (2014): 303–86.

Erenreich, Barbara, and Deirdre English, D. *For Her Own Good*. New York: Anchor Books/Doubleday, 1978.

Fagan, Robert H. "Management of the Couple with the Problem of Unsuccessful Intercourse." *Western Journal of Obstetrics and Gynecology*, 66, no. 5 (1958): 302–305.

Fahs, Breanne. *Performing Sex: The Making and Unmaking of Women's Erotic Lives*. Stony Brook, NY: SUNY Press, 2011.

Fahs, Breanne, and Eric Swank. "'The Other Third Shift?' Women's Emotion Work in Their Sexual Relationships." *Feminist Formations*, 28, no. 3 (Winter 2016): 46–69.

Fahs, Breanne, Eric Swank, and Ayanna Shambe. "'I Just Go with It': Negotiating Sexual Desire Discrepancies for Women in Partnered Relationships." *Sex Roles*, 83 (2020): 226–39.

Fenichel, Otto. *Psychoanalytic Theory of Neurosis*. New York: W. W. Norton, 1945.

Fish, Linda Stone, Ronal C. Fish, and Douglas H. Sprenkle. "Treating Inhibited Sexual Desire: A Marital Therapy Approach." *The American Journal of Family Therapy*, 12, no. 3 (January 1984): 3–12.

Foucault, Michel. "A Conversation with Michel Foucault," with John K. Simon. *Partisan Review*, 38, no. 2 (Spring 1971): 192–201.

Foucault, Michel. *The Archeology of Knowledge & the Discourse on Language*, translated by A. M. Sheridan Smith. New York: Pantheon, 1972.

Foucault, Michel. *Discipline and Punish: The Birth of the Prison*, translated by Alan Sheridan. New York: Random House, 1977.

Foucault, Michel. "Nietzsche, Genealogy, History." In *Language, Counter-Memory, Practice: Selected Essays and Interviews by Michel Foucault*, edited by Donald F. Bouchard, 139–64. Ithaca, NY: Cornell University Press, 1977.

Foucault, Michel. *The History of Sexuality: An Introduction, Vol. 1*, translated by Robert Hurley. New York: Random House, 1978.

Foucault, Michel. *Power/Knowledge: Selected Interviews and Other Writings 1972-1977*, edited by Colin Gordon, translated by Colin Gordon, Leo Marshall, John Mepham, and Kate Soper. New York: Pantheon Books, 1980.

Foucault, Michel. "The Subject of Power." *Critical Inquiry*, 8 (Summer 1982): 777–95.

Fraser, J. Scott, and Andy Solovey. "A Catalytic Approach to Sex Therapy." In *Quickies: The Handbook of Brief Sex Therapy*, edited by Shelley Green and Douglas Femmons, 189–212. New York: W. W. Norton, 2004.

Freud, Sigmund. "Fragment of an Analysis of a Case of Hysteria." In *Dora: An Analysis of a Case of Hysteria*, edited by Philip Rieff, 21–144. New York: Collier Books, 1905/1963.

Freud, Sigmund. *Three Essays on the Theory of Sexuality*, translated by James Strachey. New York: Avon Books, 1905/1962.
Freud, Sigmund. "Recommendations to Physicians Practicing Psycho-analysis." In *The Freud Reader*, edited by Peter Gay, 356–63. New York: W. W. Norton, 1912/1989.
Freud, Sigmund. *New Introductory Lectures on Psychoanalysis*, translated by James Stachey. New York: W. W. Norton, 1933.
Fricker, Miranda. *Epistemic Injustice: Power and Ethics of Knowing*. New York: Oxford University Press, 2007.
Friedan, Betty. *The Feminine Mystique*. New York: W. W. Norton, 1963.
Froman, Creel. *Language and Power, Books I & II*. Atlantic Highlands, NJ: Humanity Books, 1992.
Frost, Rebecca N., and Caroline L. Donovan. "Low Sexual Desire in Women: Amongst the Confusion Could Distress Be the Key?" *Sexual & Relationship Therapy*, 30, no. 3 (July 2015): 338–50.
Frye, Marilyn. *The Politics of Reality: Essays in Feminist Theory*. Freedom, CA: Crossing Press, 1983.
Gabbard, Glen O. Foreword. *Handbook of Sexual Dysfunction*, edited by Richard Balon and R. Taylor Segraves, iii–iv. Boca Raton, FL: Taylor & Francis, 2005.
Galinsky, Adam D., Joe C. Magee, Ena Inesi, and Deborah H. Gruenfeld. "Power and Perspectives Not Taken." *Psychological Science*, 17, no. 12 (December 2006): 1068–74.
Garfinkel, Harold. "Conditions of Successful Degradation Ceremonies." *American Journal of Sociology*, 61, no. 5 (March 1956): 420–24.
Garrigues, Henry Jacques. *A Text-Book of the Diseases of Women*. Philadelphia: W. B. Saunders, 1894.
Gavey, Nicola. "Technologies and Effects of Heterosexual Coercion." *Feminism & Psychology*, 2, no. 3 (October 1992): 325–51.
Gavey, Nicola. *Just Sex: The Cultural Scaffolding of Rape*. New York: Routledge, 2005.
Gavey, Nicola, Kathryn McPhillips, and Virginia Braun. "Interruptus Coitus: Heterosexuals Accounting for Intercourse." *Sexualities*, 2, no. 1 (February 1999): 35–68.
Gehring, Darlynne. "Couple Therapy for Low Desire: A Systemic Approach." *Journal of Sex & Marital Therapy*, 29, no. 1 (January 2003): 25–38.
Gill, Rosalind, and Rebecca Walker. "Heterosexuality, Feminism, Contradiction: On Being Young, White, Heterosexual Feminists in the 1990s." *Feminism & Psychology*, 2, no. 3 (October 1992): 453–57.
Gillett, Myrtle Mann. "Normal Frigidity in Women: A Plea to the Family Physician." *Medical Woman's Journal*, 57, no. 12 (December 1950): 29–32.
Girard, Abby, and Scott R. Wooley. "Using Emotionally Focused Therapy to Treat Sexual Desire Discrepancy in Couples." *Journal of Sex & Marital Therapy*, 43, no. 8 (November 2017): 720–35.
Goffman, Erving. *Stigma: Notes on the Management of Spoiled Identity*. Englewood Cliffs, NY: Prentice-Hall, 1963.
Goodwach, Raie. "Fundamentals of Theory and Practice Revisited: Sex Therapy: Historical Evolution, Current Practice. Part 1." *Australian and New Zealand Journal of Family Therapy*, 26, no. 3 (September 2005): 155–64.
Graber, Edward. A., Hugh K. Barber, and James J. O'Rourke. "Newlywed Apareunia." *Obstetrics & Gynecology*, 33, no. 3 (March 1969): 418–21.

Graham, Cynthia A. "Sexual Dysfunction." In *DSM-5 Clinical Cases*, edited by John W. Barnhill, 230–33, Arlington, VA: American Psychiatric Publishing, 2014.

Grayer, Justin. "Emotionally Focused Therapy for Couples: A Safe Haven from which to Explore Sex during and after Cancer." *Sexual and Relationship Therapy*, 31, no. 4 (October 2016): 488–92.

Greer, Germaine. "A Woman's Duty Is Not Only to Have Sex She Doesn't Want, But to Enjoy It." *The Times* (January 9, 2003).

Gupta, Kristina. "Compulsory Sexuality: Evaluating an Emerging Concept." *Signs: Journal of Women in Culture and Society*, 41, no. 1 (September 2015): 131–54.

Gupta, Kristina. "What Does Asexuality Teach Us about Sexual Disinterest? Recommendations for Health Professionals Based on a Qualitative Study with Asexually Identified People." *Journal of Sex & Marital Therapy*, 43, no. 1 (January 2017): 1–14.

Haden, Seymour. "The Obstetrical Society Meeting to Consider the Proposition of the Council for the Removal of Mr. I. B. Brown." *British Medical Journal*, 1, no. 327 (April 1867): 395–410.

Hall, Kathryn. "Male Hypoactive Sexual Desire Disorder." In *Systemic Sex Therapy*, edited by Katherine M. Hertlein, Gerald R. Weeks, and Nancy Gambescia, 55–71, New York: Routledge, 2015.

Hall, Marny, "Sex Therapy with Lesbian Couples: A Four Stage Approach." *Journal of Homosexuality*, 14, no. 1–2 (September 1987): 137–56.

Hall, Marny. "Not Tonight Dear, I'm Deconstructing a Headache: Confessions of a Lesbian Sex Therapist." In *A New View of Women's Sexual Problems*, edited by Ellen Kaschak and Leonore Tiefer, 161–78. New York: Haworth Press, 2001.

Hamblin, Angela. "The Suppressed Power of Female Sexuality." In *Conditions of Illusion*, edited by Sandra Allen, Lee Sanders, and Jan Wallis, 95–96. Leeds, UK: Feminist Books, 1974.

Hamilton, Eugene. G. "Frigidity in the Female." *Missouri Medicine*, 58 (October 1961): 1041–51.

Hare-Mustin, Rachel T. "Sex, Lies, and Headaches: The Problem Is Power." *Journal of Feminist Family Therapy*, 3, no. 1–2 (June 1991): 39–61.

Hare-Mustin, Rachel T. "Discourses in the Mirrored Room: A Postmodern Analysis of Therapy." *Family Process*, 33, no. 1 (March 1994): 19–35.

Hare-Mustin, Rachel T., and Jeanne Marecek. "Making a Difference." In *Making a Difference: Psychology and the Construction of Gender*, edited by Rachel T. Hare-Mustin and Jeanne Marecek, 1–21. New Haven, CT: Yale University Press, 1990.

Harmon, Marsha J., Michael Waldo, and James A. Johnson. "Relationship Enhancement Therapy: A Case Study for Treatment of Vaginismus." *The Family Journal*, 2, no. 2 (April 1994): 122–28.

Hartman, William E., and Marilyn A. Fithian. "A Non-Orgasmic Women Study." Paper presented to the National Council on Family Relations Annual Meeting, New Orleans, October 1968.

Hartman, William E., and Marilyn A. Fithian. "Sexual Myths." *Family Court Review*, 9, no. 1 (September 1971): 19–24.

Hartman, William E., and Marilyn A. Fithian. *Treatment of Sexual Dysfunction: A Bio-Psycho-Social Approach*. Long Beach, CA: Center for Marital and Sexual Studies, 1972.

Hartman, William E., and Marilyn A. Fithian. "Additional Comment on the Sexological Exam: A Reply to Hoch." *Journal of Sex Research*, 18, no. 1 (February 1982): 64–71.

Hartogs, Renatus. "Analyst's Couch." *Cosmopolitan* (November 1969), 60.
Hayles, N. Katherine. "Anger in Different Voices: Carol Gilligan and 'The Mill on the Floss.'" *Signs*, 12, no. 1 (October 1986): 23–39.
Hendrickx, Lies, Luk Gijs, and Paul Enzlin. "Prevalence Rates of Sexual Difficulties and Associated Distress in Heterosexual Men and Women: Results from an Internet Survey in Flanders." *Journal of Sex Research*, 51, no. 1 (January 2013): 1–12.
Herbenick, Debby, Margo Mullinax, and Kristen Mark. "Sexual Desire Discrepancy as a Feature, Not a Bug, of Long-Term Relationships." *Journal of Sexual Medicine*, 11, no. 9 (September 2014). 2196–2206.
Herman, Judith L. *Trauma and Recovery: The Aftermath of Violence from Domestic Abuse to Political Terror*. New York: Basic Books, 1992.
Hite, Shere. *The Hite Report: A National Study of Female Sexuality*. New York: Seven Stories Press, 2004.
Hite, Shere. *The Shere Hite Reader: New and Selected Writings on Sex, Globalism, and Private Life*. New York: Seven Stories Press, 2011.
Hitschmann, Eduard, and Edmund Bergler. *Frigidity in Women: Its Characteristics and Treatment*. New York: Nervous and Mental Disease Publishing, 1936.
Hitschmann, Eduard, and Edmund Bergler. "Frigidity in Women—Restatement and Renewed Experiences." *Psychoanalytic Review*, 36, no. 1 (1949): 45–53.
Hochschild, Arlie. *The Managed Heart: Commercialization of Human Feeling*. Berkeley, CA: University of California Press, 1983.
Hochschild, Arlie, and Anne Machung. *The Second Shift: Working Families and the Revolution at Home*. New York: Penguin, 2012.
Hunter, John. *Treatise on Venereal Disease*. London: Leicester-Square, 1786.
Iasenza, Suzanne. "Multicontextual Sex Therapy with Lesbian Couples." In *Quickies: The Handbook of Brief Sex Therapy*, edited by Shelley Green and Jennifer Hornsby, 15–25. New York: W. W. Norton, 2004.
Implett, Emily. A., and Letitia Anne Peplau. "Why Some Women Consent to Unwanted Sex with a Dating Partner: Insights from Attachment Theory." *Psychology of Women Quarterly*, 26, no. 4 (December 2002): 360–70.
Irvine, Janice M. *Disorders of Desire: Sexuality and Gender in Modern American Sexology*. Philadelphia: Temple University Press, 2005.
Jackson, Margaret. "Sex Research and the Construction of Sexuality: A Tool of Male Supremacy?" *Women's Studies Int. Forum*, 7, no. 1 (January 1984): 43–51.
Jackson, Stevi, and Sue Scott. "Embodying Orgasm: Gendered Power Relations and Sexual Pleasure." In *A New View of Women's Sexual Problems*, edited by Ellen Kaschak and Leonore Tiefer, 99–110. New York: Haworth Press, 2012.
Janata, Jeffry W., and Sheryl A. Kingsberg. "Sexual Aversion Disorder." In *Handbook of Sexual Dysfunction*, edited by Richard Balon and R. Taylor Segraves, 111–21. Boca Raton, FL: Taylor & Francis, 2005.
Jenkins, David, and Lon Johnston. "Unethical Treatment of Gay and Lesbian People with Conversion Therapy." *Families in Society: The Journal of Contemporary Social Services*, 84, no. 4 (January 2004): 557–61.
Jernigan, Lindsay B. "Compassionate Authenticity: A Treatment Model for Working with Women with Low Libido." *Sexual and Relationship Therapy*, 29, no. 1 (January 2014): 56–67.
Johnston, Dusty J. "A Listening Guide Analysis of Women's Experiences of Unacknowledged Rape." *Psychology of Women Quarterly*, 40, no. 2 (June 2016): 275–89.

Jung, Carl. *Memories, Dreams, Reflections*, translated by Richard and Clara Winston. London: Random House, 1963.

Kahane, Claire. "Why Dora Now? (Introduction, Part 2)." In *Dora's Case: Freud—Hysteria—Feminism*, edited by Carles Bernheimer and Claire Kahane, 19–32. New York: Columbia University Press, 1985.

Kaplan, Helen Singer. *The New Sex Therapy: Active Treatment of Sexual Dysfunctions*. New York: Times Books, 1974.

Kaplan, Helen Singer. *Disorders of Sexual Desire and Other New Concepts and Techniques in Sex Therapy*. New York: Brunner/Mazel, 1979.

Kaplan, Helen Singer. *Sexual Aversion, Sexual Phobias, and Panic Disorders*. New York: Brunner/Mazel, 1987.

Kaplan, Helen Singer. *The Sexual Desire Disorders: Dysfunctional Regulation of Sexual Motivation*. New York: Brunner/Mazel, 1995.

Katz, Jonathan Ned. *The Invention of Heterosexuality*. New York: Dutton, 1995.

Kazin, Alfred. "The Freudian Revolution Analyzed." In *Freud and the Twentieth Century*, edited by Benjamin Nelso, 13–21. Gloucester, MA: Peter Smith, 1957.

Kessler, Jo Marie. "When the Diagnosis Is Vaginismus: Fighting Misconceptions." *Women & Therapy*, 7, no. 2-3 (1988): 175–86.

Kinsey, Alfred C., Wardell B. Pomeroy, and Paul H. Gebhard. *Sexual Behavior in the Human Female*. Philadelphia: W. B. Saunders, 1953.

Kleinplatz, Peggy J. "Sex Therapy for Vaginismus: A Review, Critique, and Humanistic Alternative." *Journal of Humanistic Psychology*, 38, no. 2 (April 1998): 51–81.

Kleinplatz, Peggy, J. "History of the Treatment of Female Sexual Dysfunction(s)." *Annual Review of Clinical Psychology*, 14, no. 1 (May 2018): 29–54.

Koedt, Anne. "The Myth of the Vaginal Orgasm." In *Radical Feminism*, edited by Anne Koedt, Ellen Levine, and Anita Rapone, 198–207. New York: Quadrangle Books, 1973.

Koss, Mary P. "Hidden, Unacknowledged, Acquaintance, and Date Rape: Looking Back, Looking Forward." *Psychology of Women Quarterly*, 35, no. 2 (June 2011): 348–54.

Koss, Mary P., Christine A Gidycz, and Nadine Wisniewski, N. "The Scope of Rape: Incidence and Prevalence of Sexual Aggression and Victimization in a National Sample of Higher Education Students." *Journal of Consulting & Clinical Psychology*, 55, no. 2 (April 1987): 162–70.

Krasnow, Stefanie Sara, and Asa-Sophia Maglio. "Female Sexual Desire: What Helps, What Hinders, and What Women Want." *Sexual and Relationship Therapy* (2019). doi:10.1080/14681994.2019.1626011.

Kroger, William S., and S. Charles Freed. "Psychosomatic Aspects of Frigidity." *Journal of the American Medical Association*, 143, no. 6 (June 1950): 526–32.

Kroger, William S., and S. Charles Freed. *Psychosomatic Gynecology*. Philadelphia: Saunders, 1951.

Kuhn, Thomas. *The Structure of Scientific Revolutions*. Chicago: University of Chicago Press, 1970.

Langton, Rae. "Feminism in Epistemology: Exclusion and Objectification." In *The Cambridge Companion to Feminism in Philosophy*, edited by Marilyn Fricker and Jennifer Hornsby, 127–45. Cambridge, UK: Cambridge University Press, 2000.

Lazarus, Arnold A. "The Treatment of Chronic Frigidity by Systematic Desensitization." *Journal of Nervous and Mental Disease*, 131, no. 3 (March 1963): 272–78.

Leaiblum, Sandra, R. "Preface." In *Principles and Practice of Sex Therapy*, edited by Sandra R. Leiblum, xi–xiii. New York: Guilford, 2007.

Leiblum, Sandra R., Lawrence A. Pervin, and Enid H. Campbell. "The Treatment of Vaginismus: Success and Failure." In *Principles and Practice of Sex Therapy*, edited by Sandra R. Leiblum and Raymond C. Rosen, 113–38. New York: Guilford, 1989.

Lev, Arlene Istar, and Margaret Nichols. "Sex Therapy with Lesbian and Gay Couples." In *Systemic Sex Therapy*, edited by Katherine M. Hertlein, Gerald R. Weeks, and Nancy Gambescio, 213–34. New York: Routledge, 2015.

Lief, Harold I. "Integrative Therapy in a Woman with Secondary Low Sex Drive." In *Case Studies in Sex Therapy*, edited by Raymond C. Rosen and Sandra R. Leiblum, 110–30. New York: Guilford, 1995.

LoPicollo, Joseph. "Masters Series." American Association of Marriage and Family Therapists, Videotape, October 1989.

Lundberg, Ferdinand, and Marynia F. Farnham. *Modern Woman: The Lost Sex*. New York: Harper & Brothers, 1947.

Lydon, Susan. *The Politics of Orgasm*. New York: Vintage Books, Random House, 1970.

MacKinnon, Catharine A. *Sexual Harassment of Working Women: A Case of Discrimination*. New Haven, CT: Yale University Press, 1979.

MacKinnon, Catharine A. *Feminism Unmodified: Discourses on Life and Law*. Cambridge, MA: Harvard University Press, 1987.

MacKinnon, Catharine A. "Rape Redefined." *Harvard Law & Policy Review*, 10 (2016): 431–77.

Macmillan, Malcolm. *Freud Evaluated: The Completed Arc*. Amsterdam, The Netherlands: Elsevier, 1991.

Maddon, Thomas More. "The Treatment of Vaginismus." *Dublin Journal of Medical Science*, 83, no. 2 (February 1887): 129–34.

Mahoney, Patrick. *Freud's Dora: A Psychoanalytic, Historical, and Textual Study*. New Haven, CT: Yale University Press, 1996.

Malcolm, Janet. *Psychoanalysis: The Impossible Profession*. London, UK: Karmac, 1982.

Malleson, Joan. "Sex Problems in Marriage with Particular Reference to Coital Discomfort and the Unconsummated Marriage." *The Practitioner*, 172, no. 1030 (April 1954): 389–96.

Manne, Kate. *Down Girl: The Logic of Misogyny*. Oxford, UK: Oxford University Press, 2018.

Marcus, Steven. "Freud and Dora: Story, History, Case History." In *Dora's Case: Freud—Hysteria—Feminism*, edited by Charles Bernheimer and Claire Kahane, 56–91. New York: Columbia University Press, 1985.

Margolin, Leslie. "Dilators, Q-tips, and Extortion: How to Train a Woman for Intercourse in the 'Post-Feminist' Era." *Journal of Feminist Family Therapy*, 29, no. 4 (October 2017): 189–204.

Margolin, Leslie. "Freud, Dora, and Compulsory Sexuality." *Journal of Humanistic Psychology* (2017). doi:10.1177/0022167817739744

Margolin, Leslie. "Sexual Frigidity: The Social Construction of Masculine Privilege and Feminine Pathology." *Journal of Gender Studies*, 26, no. 5 (Sept. 2017): 583–94.

Masters, William H., and Virginia E. Johnson. *Human Sexual Response*. Boston: Little, Brown, 1966.

Masters, William H., and Virginia E. Johnson. "Playboy Interview: Masters and Johnson." In *Masters and Johnson Explained*, edited by Nat Lerman, 128–72. Chicago: Playboy Press, 1968.

Masters, William H., and Virginia E. Johnson. *Human Sexual Inadequacy*. Boston: Little, Brown, 1970.

Masters, William H., and Virginia E. Johnson. *The Pleasure Bond: A Look at Sexuality and Commitment*. Boston: Little, Brown, 1970.

Masters, William H., and Virginia E. Johnson. "Principles of the New Sex Therapy." *American Journal of Psychiatry*, 133, no. 5 (May 1976): 548–54.

Maurice, William L. "Sexual Desire Disorders in Men." In *Principles and Practice of Sex Therapy*, 4th ed., edited by Sandra R. Leiblum, 181–211. New York: Guilford, 2007.

May, Elaine Tyler. *Homeward Bound: American Families in the Cold War Era*. New York: Basic Books, 2008.

McClelland, Sara I. "Who is the 'Self' in Self-Reports of Sexual Satisfaction? Research and Policy Implications." *Sexuality Research and Social Policy*, 8, no. 4 (December 2011): 304–20.

McCormick, Naomi B. *Sexual Salvation: Affirming Women's Sexual Rights and Pleasures*. Westport, CT: Praeger, 1994.

Meadmore, Dapne, Caroline Hatcher, and Erica McMillen. "Getting Tense about Genealogy." *International Journal of Qualitative Studies about Education*, 13, no. 5 (September 2000): 463–76.

Meana, Marta. "Elucidating Women's (Hetero)Sexual Desire: Definitional Challenges and Content Expansion." *Journal of Sex Research*, 47, no. 2–3 (March 2010): 104–22.

Meana, Marta, Evan Fertel, and Caroline Maykut. "Treating Genital Pain Associated with Intercourse." In *The Wiley Handbook of Sex Therapy*, edited by Zoe Peterson, 98–114. Malden, MA: Wiley, 2017.

Meana, Marta, and Eric T. Steiner. "Hidden Disorder/Hidden Desire: Presentations of Low Sexual Desire in Men." In *Principles and Practice of Sex Therapy*, 5th ed., edited by Yitzchak M. Binik and Kathryn S. K. Hall, 42–60. New York: Guilford, 2014.

Miller, Scott D., Karen M. Donahey, and Mark A. Hubble. "Getting 'in the Mood' (for a Change): Stage-appropriate Clinical Work for Sexual Problems." In *Quickies: The Handbook for Brief Sex Therapy*, edited by Shelley Green and Douglas Flemmons, 26–44. New York: W.W. Norton, 2004.

Millett, Kate. *Sexual Politics*. New York: Doubleday, 1970.

Moi, Toril. "Representations of Patriarchy: Sexuality and Epistemology in Freud's Dora." In *Dora's Case: Freud—Hysteria—Feminism*, edited Charles Bernheimer and Claire Kahane, 181–99. New York: Columbia University Press, 1985.

Morber, Jenny. "What Science Says about Arousal during Rape: Yes, Orgasms Can Happen to Rape Victims," May 30, 2013: http://www.popscie.com/science/article/2013-2015/science-arousal-during-rape.

Morton, Thomas. G. "Removal of the Ovaries as a Cure for Insanity." *American Journal of Psychiatry*, 49, no. 3 (January 1893): 391–96.

Morrison, Toni. *The Bluest Eye*. New York: Holt, Rinehart, and Winston, 1970.

Morrow, Ross. *Sex Research and Sex Therapy: A Sociological Analysis of Masters and Johnson*. New York: Routledge, 2013.

Muehlenhard, Charlene L., and Sheena K. Shippee. "Men's and Women's Reports of Pretending Orgasm." *Journal of Sex Research*, 47, no. 6 (November 2010): 552–67.

Nichols, Margaret, and Michael Shernoff. "Therapy with Sexual Minorities: Queering Practice." In *Principles and Practice of Sex Therapy*, 4th ed., edited by Sandra R. Leiblum, 379–415. New York: Guilford, 2007.

Nicholson, Paula, and Jennifer Burr. "'What Is 'Normal' about Women's (Hetero)Sexual Desire and Orgasm?' A Report of an In-Depth Interview Study." *Social Science & Medicine* 57, no. 9 (November 2003): 1735–45.

Orwell, George. *1984.* New York: New American Library, 1949.
Pertot, Sandra. *Perfectly Normal: Living and Loving with Low Libido.* New York: Rosedale, 2005.
Peterson, Zoe O., and Charlene L. Muehlenhard. "Conceptualizing the 'Wantedness' of Women's Consensual and Nonconsensual Sexual Experiences: Implications for How Women Label Their Experiences with Rape." *Journal of Sex Research,* 44, no. 1 (April 2007): 72–88.
Phillips, Kathryn, Virginia Braun, and Nicola Gavet. "Defining (Hetero)Sex: How Imperative Is the Coital Imperative?" Women's Studies International Form, 24, no. 2 (March-April 2001): 229–40.
Pietsch, Ursula K. "Strategic Treatment of Female Hypoactive Sexual Desire Disorder." *Journal of Family Psychotherapy,* 12, no. 4 (December 2001): 31–44.
Pollner, Melvin. *Mundane Reason: Reality in Everyday and Sociological Discourse.* Cambridge, UK: Cambridge University Press, 1987.
Potts, Annie. "Coming, Coming, Gone: A Feminist Deconstruction of Heterosexual Orgasm." *Sexualities,* 3, no. 1 (February 2000): 55–76.
Potts, Annie. *The Science/Fiction of Sex: Feminist Deconstruction and the Vocabularies of Heterosex.* New York: Routledge, 2002.
Regas, Susan J., and Douglas H. Sprenkle. "Functional Family Therapy and the Treatment of Inhibited Sexual Desire." *Journal of Marital and Family Therapy,* 10, no. 1 (January 1984): 63–72.
Reissing, Elke D., Yitzchak M. Binik, and Samir Khalife. "Does Vaginismus Exist: A Critical Review of the Literature." *The Journal of Nervous & Mental Disease,* 187, no. 5 (May 1999): 261–74.
Renshaw, Domeena C. "Sexless Marriages and Sex Therapy." In *Case Studies in Sex Therapy,* edited by Raymond C. Rosen and Sandra R. Leiblum, 176–89. New York: Guilford, 1995.
Rhode, Deborah L. *Speaking of Sex: The Denial of Gender Inequality.* Cambridge, MA: Harvard University Press, 1999.
Rich, Adrienne. *Of Woman Born: Motherhood as Experience and Institution.* New York: W.W. Norton, 1986.
Richgels, Patricia B. "Hypoactive Sexual Desire in Heterosexual Women: A Feminist Analysis." *Women & Therapy,* 12, no. 1–2 (September 1992): 123–35.
Robinson, Marie Nyswander. *The Power of Sexual Surrender.* New York: Doubleday, 1959.
Robinson, William Josephus. *Married Life and Happiness: Or, Love and Comfort in Marriage.* New York: Eugenics Publishing, 1922.
Rosen, Raymond C., and Sandra R Leiblum. "Assessment and Treatment of Desire Disorders." In *Principles and Practice of Sex Therapy,* 2nd ed., edited by Sandra R. Leiblum and Raymond C. Rosen, 19–47. New York: Guilford, 1989.
Rosen, Raymond C., and Sandra R. Leiblum. Preface to *Case Studies in Sex Therapy,* edited by Raymond C. Rosen and Sandra R. Leiblum, ix–xi. New York: Guillford, 1995.
Rosen, Raymond C., Jan L. Shifren, Brigitta U. Monz, Dawn Odom, Patricia A. Russo, and Catherine B. Johannes. "Epidemiology: Correlates of Sexually Related Personal Distress in Women with Low Sexual Desire." *The Journal of Sexual Medicine,* 6, no. 6 (June 2009): 1549–1560.
Sanchez, Diane T., Amy K. Kiefer, and Oscar Ybarro. "Sexual Submissiveness in Women: Costs for Sexual Autonomy and Arousal." *Sexual and Relationship Therapy,* 27, no. 4 (April 2006): 344–57.

Schwartz, Mark. F., and Masters, William. H. "Inhibited Sexual Desire: The Masters and Johnson Treatment Model." In *Sexual Desire Disorders*, edited by Sandra R. Leiblum and Raymond C. Rosen, 229–42. New York: Guilford, 1988.

Sedgwick, Eve Kosofsky. *The Epistemology of the Closet*. Berkeley, CA: University of California Press, 1990.

Shaw, Jeanne. "The Treatment of Vaginismus: What Is Wrong with this Picture?" Paper presented at SSTAR Annual Meeting, Redondo Beach, CA, March 1991.

Shaw, Jeanne. "Treatment of Primary Vaginismus: A New Perspective." *Journal of Sex & Marital Therapy*, 20, no. 1 (March 1994): 46–55.

Shifren, Jan L., Brigitta U. Monz, Patricia A. Russo, Anthony A. Segreti, and Catherine B. Johannes. "Sexual Problems and Distress in United States Women: Prevalence and Correlates." *Obstetrics & Gynecology*, 112, no. 5 (November 2008): 970–78.

Sims, James Marion. *Clinical Notes on Women's Surgery: With Reference to the Management of the Sterile Condition*. New York: William Wood & Co., 1866.

Spitzer, Robert L. "The Diagnostic Status of Homosexuality in *DSM-III*: A Reformulation of the Issues." *American Journal of Psychiatry*, 138, no. 2 (February 1981): 210–15.

Spitzer, Robert, L., Jean Endicott, and Jean-Arthur Micoulaud Franchi. "Medical and Mental Disorder: Proposed Definition and Criteria." *Annales Medico-Psychologiques*, 178, no. 7 (September 2018): 656–65.

Spitzer, Robert, L., Miriam Gibbon, Andrew E. Skodol, Janet B. W. Williams, and Michael B. First. *DSM-III-R Case Book: A Learning Companion to the Diagnostic and Statistical Manual of Mental Disorders*, 3rd ed., revised. Washington, DC: American Psychiatric Press, 1989.

Spitzer, Robert L., Miriam Gibbon, Andrew E. Skodol, Janet B. W. Williams, and Michael B. First. *DSM-IV Case Book: A Learning Companion to the Diagnostic and Statistical Manual of Mental Disorders*, 4th edition. Washington, DC: American Psychiatric Press, 1994.

Spitzer, Robert L., Miriam Gibbon, Andrew E. Skodol, Janet B. W. Williams, and Michael B. First. *DSM-IV-TR Case Book: A Learning Companion to the Diagnostic and Statistical Manual of Mental Disorders*, 4th edition, text revision, Washington, DC: American Psychiatric Publishing, 2002. https://www.petertatchell.net/lgbt_rights/psychiatry/freud/

Spitzer, Robert L., Andrew E. Skodol, Miriam Gibbon, and Janet B. W. Williams (eds.). *DSM-III Case Book: A Learning Companion to the Diagnostic and Statistical Manual of Mental Disorders*, 3rd ed. Washington, DC: American Psychiatric Association, 1981.

Stekel, Wilhelm. *Frigidity in Woman in Relation to Her Love Life*. New York: Liveright, 1943.

Stephenson, Kyle R., and Cindy M. Weston. "Consequences of Impaired Female Sexual Functioning: Individual Differences and Associations with Sexual Distress." *Sexual and Relationship Therapy*, 27, no. 1 (November 2012): 344–57.

Stone, Hannah M., and Abraham Stone. *A Marriage Manual*. New York: Simon & Schuster, 1937.

Tatchell, Peter. "Freud and the Liberation of Sexual Desire," 1989 https://www.petertatchell.net/lgbt_rights/psychiatry/freud/

Tiefer, Leonore. *Sex Is Not a Natural Act & Other Essays*. Boulder, CO: Westview Press, 1995.

Tiefer, Leonore. "The Social Construction and Social Effects of Sex Research: The Sexological Model of Sexuality." In *Sexuality, Society, and Feminism*, edited by

Cheryl Brown Travis and Jacqueline W. White, 79–107. Washington, DC: American Psychological Association, 2000.

Tiefer, Leonore. "Feminist Critique of Sex Therapy: Foregrounding the Politics of Sex." In *New Directions in Sex Therapy: Innovations and Alternatives*, edited by Peggy J. Kleinplatz, 29–49. Philadelphia: Brunner-Routledge, 2001.

Tiefer, Leonore. "A 'New View' Campaign: A Feminist Critique of Sex Therapy and an Alternative Vision." In *New Directions in Sex Therapy: Innovations and Alternatives* edited by Peggy J. Kleinplatz, 21–35. Hoboken, NJ: Taylor & Francis, 2012.

Tiefer, Leonore and 21 others. Letter to FDA regarding Docket No. 00D: 1278, Draft Guidance: Female Sexual Dysfunction: Clinical Development of Drug Products for Treatment. Mailed in two parts, June 19, 2000 (12 co-signers), and July 10, 2000 (9 co-signers).

Torres, M. Gabriella. "Reconciling Cultural Difference in the Study of Marital Rape." In *Marital Rape: Consent, Marriage, and Social Change in Global Context*, edited by Kersti Yllo and M. Gabriella Torres, 9–17. Oxford, UK: Oxford University Press, 2016.

Torres, M. Gabriella, and Yllo, Kersti. "Implications for Policy, Practice, and Future Research." In *Marital Rape: Consent, Marriage, and Social Change in Global Context*, edited by Kersti Yllo and M. Gabriella Torres, 199–203. Oxford, UK: Oxford University Press, 2016.

Tuana, Nancy. "The Speculum of Ignorance: The Women's Health Movement and Epistemologies of Ignorance." *Hypatia*, 21, no. 3 (August 2006): 1–19.

Van de Velde, Theodore H. *Ideal Marriage: Its Physiology and Technique*. New York: Random House, 1926.

Ventura, Elizabeth (ed.). *Casebook for DSM-5: Diagnosis and Treatment Planning*, New York: Springer, 2017.

Weeks, Gerald R., Katherine M. Hertlein, and Nancy Gambesci. Preface to *Systemic Sex Therapy*, edited by Gerald R. Weeks, Katherine M. Hertlein, and Nancy Gambesci. xxiv–xxix, New York: Routledge, 2015.

Weiner, M. F. Wives Who Refuse Their Husbands." Psychosomatics, 14, no. 5 (1973): 277–282.

West, Robin. "Equality Theory, Marital Rape, and the Promise of the Fourteenth Amendment." *Florida Law Review*, 42 (1990): 45–79.

West, Robin. "The Harms of Consensual Sex." In *The Philosophy of Sex: Contemporary Readings*, edited by Raja Halwani, Alan Sobel, Sarah Hoffman, and Jacob M. Held, 371–80. London: Rowan & Littlefield, 2017.

West, Suzanne. L., Aimee A. D'Aloisio, Robert P. Agans, William D. Kalsbeek, Natalie N. Borisov, and John M. Thorp. "Prevalence of Low Sexual Desire and Hypoactive Sexual Desire in a Nationally Representative Sample of US Women." *Archives of Internal Medicine*, 168, no. 13 (July 2008): 1441–49.

Wiederman, Michael W. "Pretending Orgasm During Sexual Intercourse: Correlates in a Sample of Young Adult Women." *Journal of Marital & Sex Therapy*, 23, no. 2 (June 1997): 131–39.

Wijma, Barbro, and Klass Wijma. "A Cognitive Behavioural Treatment Model of Vaginismus." *Scandinavian Journal of Behavioural Therapy*, 26, no. 4 (October 1997): 147–56.

Willyard, Cassandra. "Men: A Growing Minority?" January 2011: https://www.apa.org/gradpsych/2011/01/cover-men

Wilson, Mitchell. "DSM-III and the Transformation of American Psychiatry: A History." *American Journal of Psychiatry*, 150, no. 3 (March 1993): 399–410.

Wittgenstein, Ludwig. "Conversations on Freud." In *Wittgenstein: Lectures and Conversations: On Aesthetics, Psychology, and Religious Belief*, edited by Cyril Barrett, 42–52. Oxford, UK: Basil Blackwell & Mott, 1966.

Wolpe, Joseph. *Psychotherapy by Reciprocal Inhibition*. Stanford, CA: Stanford University Press, 1958.

Wolpe, Joseph. *The Practice of Behavior Therapy*. New York: Pergamon Press, 1968.

Wolpe, Joseph. "The Treatment of Inhibited Sexual Responses." In *Handbook of Behavior Therapy with Sexual Problems, Volume 1: General Procedures*, edited by Joel Fischer and Harvey L. Gochoros, 46–58. New York: Pergamon Press, 1977.

Woo, Elaine. "Marilyn Fithian Obituary," *Los Angeles Times*, September 19, 2008.

Wortis, Joseph. "Fragments of a Freudian Analysis." *American Journal of Orthopsychiatry*, 10, no. 4 (October 1940): 843–49.

Wylie, Kevan R., Desa Markovic, and Ruth Hallam-Jones. "Inhibited Arousal in Women." In *Systemic Sex Therapy*, edited by Katherine M. Hertlein, Gerald R. Weeks, and Nancy Gambescia, 152–70. New York: Routledge, 2015.

Young, Sarah, "Three Quarters of People Cannot Define Asexuality." *Independent* (Feb. 3, 2019): https://www.independent.co.uk/life-style/asexual-meaning-definition-what-is-asexuality-sky-poll-a8760826.html.

Zussman, L., Zussman, S., Ellison, C., Salzman, L., and Sorg, D. A. (1974). "Treatment of a Case of Vaginal Constriction Preventing Coitus." *Medical Aspects of Human Sexuality*, 8, 80–109.

Index

For the benefit of digital users, indexed terms that span two pages (e.g., 52–53) may, on occasion, appear on only one of those pages.

adaptation of woman to man's desires
   free will of men, 131, 136n.43, 126–34
   woman's duty, 140–42
Antony, Louise, 175
asexuality, 4, 9n.45, 31
automanipulative techniques. *See* masturbation

Barry, Kathleen, 73
Basson, Rosemary, 167n.2
Bauer, Ida. *See* Dora case study
behavioral sex therapy, 12
Bergler, Edmund, 32–33, 34–35, 36–37, 38–40, 41, 42–43, 44, 50
biopsychosocial approach
   accusation of collusion, 103–4
   anxiety hierarchy of scenes, 100–2
   devaluation of wife's testimony, 96–97
   Hartman/Fithian principles, 91, 92
   husband's behaviors/wife's disinterest, 94–97
   intercourse as prescription, 104n.46, 102–5, 125–26
   intercourse imperative, 100n.36, 100–2
   motivations for sex, 98–99
   motivations to seek treatment, 96–97
   normal sexual response development, 94n.25
   organization, men *vs.* women, 97–98
   sex as ownership of woman, 89–90n.4
   systematic desensitization, 92–100
   vagina, focus on, 91–92n.10
   vaginismus, 99–100, 104n.46, 102–5
   woman's responsiveness, 88–90
   women's exercises, 92n.10
blaming of women
   frigidity theory, 38–41

frigidity theory, blame shifting by women, 39–40
intercourse imperative, 5–7n.30
male identification, 80–81, 83–84
orgasm, lack of, 113
Blank, Hanne, 4n.14
body/mind awareness building, 158–60
Bonaparte, Marie, 38

Caprio, Frank S., 32, 39, 44
case studies
   Adam/Jen, 161–63
   Alice, 139
   Anna/Derek, 157–58
   arranged/forced marriage, 85–87
   A's, 92–100
   Bill/Belle, 125–26, 153–54
   Brad/Lisa, 145–47n.44
   Brad/Stacey, 135
   B's, 110–12n.7
   Caroline, 114–15n.18, 115–18n.23, 119, 125–26
   Chris/Sarah, 149–50
   Dave/Alicia, 127–29, 131
   Dawn/Tim, 132–34
   Deb/Ron, 134–36
   Dora (*see* Dora case study)
   D's, 142–43
   Edward/Jocelyn, 156–57
   Elizabeth/Finn, 163–65
   Esther/Shlomo, 85–87
   female orgasmic disorder, 112–13, 138–42, 151
   Francis, 160–61
   Holt, Nancy, 75–76, 128
   Jamie/Sheila, 148–50
   Jan/Sue, 153–54
   Joe, 76–79

case studies (*cont.*)
   Joyce/Bill, 143–45
   Kari/Greg, 139–40, 150–51
   Laura, 112–13
   Lil, 119–21, 127
   Liz/Scottie, 152–53
   Luz, 111–12n.8
   Marie/Paul, 129
   Mary, 138–42, 151–52
   methodology, 8–10
   Mrs. A., 93–98
   M's, 82–84, 87
   Nadia/Ivan, 129–32, 145
   Norma/Norman, 74–76, 79
   Patricia/Edward, 158–60
   Sam/Jo, 151–52
   Susan/Nick, 126–32, 135
catarrh (leucorrhoea), 28–29
Chideckel, Maurice, 37, 43
chimney sweeping technique, 123
Clark, LeMon, 155
cliteridectomy, 2–3n.4
clitoridal woman, 37
clitoris in pathological inhibition, 37
Coetzee, J. M., 1
coital imperative, 4n.13.
   See also intercourse imperative
Cole, William Graham, 21
compulsory sexuality. *See* Dora case study
consent to sex by women
   enjoyment *vs.*, 115–16n.18, 115–16n.20
   free will of women, 130–32
   husband's frustration, 111n.7
   intercourse imperative, 5n.17, 53, 56
   male identification, 76
   power relationships, 53, 56
   sex therapy reform, 176
   sexual dysfunctions, 111–12n.8
Copley, Sanford, 64n.60

Dahl, Robert, 54–55
Densmore, Dana, 50
Dickinson, Robert Latou, 38
dismissal of woman's perspective
   Dora case study, 24
   free will of men, 131–34
   sex therapy reform, 175–77
   sexual dysfunctions, 123
   woman's duty, 138–40

Donovan, Caroline L., 136
Dora case study
   birth of, 23n.14
   children's bed-wetting, 28–29
   compulsory sexuality, 22
   dismissal of Dora's perspective, 24, 25–26, 29, 31
   dream interpretation, 26–28
   Freud's concept of sexuality, 21n.3, 64
   Freud's domination, 148
   Freud's sexual fixations, 22, 23–24n.17, 23–26, 30–31
   Freud's talking cure, 22–23
   jewel-case symbolism, 27
   lack of assent/denial of attraction, 24, 25–26, 27–28, 29, 64, 73, 148
   letter/secret symbolism, 30
   masturbation interpretation, 28–31
   oral sex fixation, 24–25
   overview, 23
   parent's extramarital affair, 24–25
   reticule, 29–30
   sexual abuse, Dora's reaction to, 23–24
   sexual discrepancy, 11
   symptom as sexual fantasy, 24–25
   tacit acceptance of unconscious desire, 24–26
double consciousness, 132–34
DSM III, 12, 109–10
DSM-IV/DSM-5, 13, 163
Du Bois, W. E. B., 132
duty. *See* woman's duty
Dworkin, Andrea, 4, 7, 17, 77, 90n.4, 142

Elliott, Sinikka, 115–16n.20, 145
Ellis, Havelock, 38
emotional connection, building, 161–63, 176
equivalency myth, 77n.17, 74–76
etherization during sex, 1–2

Fagan, Robert H., 32–33n.7
Fahs, Breanne, 77
Farnham, Marynia F., 21n.3, 37
female hypoactive desire disorder, 156–57
female orgasmic disorder, 112–13, 138–42, 151
female sexual interest/desire disorder, 163–64

INDEX   221

Fenichel, Otto, 3
Fithian, Marilyn, 12, 91, 92n.10, 92n.14,
    100n.36. *See also* biopsychosocial
    approach
Foucault, Michel, 10–11, 16–17, 21,
    93–94, 156
free will of men
    adaptation of woman to man's desires,
       131, 136n.43, 126–34
    dismissal of woman's
       perspective, 131–34
    double consciousness, 132–34
    low sexual desire/man, 125–26,
       134–36
    low sexual desire/woman, 129–34
    male frigidity, 127–29
    man's insecurities *vs.* woman's
       neuroses, 139–40
    therapy challenges, 134–36
Freud, Sigmund, 3, 11, 21–23n.3,
    23–24n.17, 33, 50, 64–67, 123.
    See also Dora case study
Fricker, Miranda, 16–17
Friedan, Betty, 46
frigidity theory
    blame shifting by women, 39–40
    blaming of women, 38–41
    concepts, definitions, 34–36
    diagnosis, 34–36, 37, 49
    fall of, 49–50
    Freudian concepts of, 33
    hatred of men, 43–44
    husband's behaviors/wife's disinterest,
       33, 38–40, 62
    male impotence, 38–40
    measurement of, 41–44
    normal women ideal, 11–12, 44–46
    power relationships, 32–33n.7,
       34–36n.25
    premature ejaculation, 34–35
    sexual abuse by therapist, 35–36n.25
    sexual energy flow theory, 32–33
    successful intercourse factors, 32–33n.7
    women's neuroses in, 33, 35, 36–37
Frost, Rebecca N., 136
Frye, Marilyn, 16–17, 173

Garrigues, Henry J., 2–3n.4
Gavey, Nicola, 14–15n.62

gender differences in sexual desire,
    6–7n.30
gender imperialism, 4n.12
gender inequality, Kaplan on, 74
genealogical history, 10–11
Gill, Rosalind, 71
Gillett, Mary Mann, 33
Goffman, Erving, 171
Greer, Germaine, 155, 175

Haden, Seymour, 11n.51
Hall, Marny, 65, 148
Hamilton, E. G., 44, 45
Hare-Mustin, Rachel, 16, 165
Hartman, William, 12, 91, 92n.10,
    100n.36. *See also* biopsychosocial
    approach
Hayles, Katherine, 85–86
Hite, Shere, 5n.17, 7n.31, 64n.60, 71–72
Hitschmann, Eduard, 32–33, 34, 35, 36–
    37, 41, 42–43, 44
Hochschild, Arlie, 69n.75, 75–76
homosexuality as psychiatric disorder,
    109. *See also* lesbian couples
HSD (hypoactive sexual desire),
    81–85, 99n.34
Hunter, John, 69n.75
husband's behaviors/wife's disinterest
    biopsychosocial approach, 94–97
    forced intercourse, 145–47n.44
    frigidity theory, 33, 38–40, 62
    woman's duty, 140–41, 143–47n.44

impaired functioning in diagnosis, 168–69
impotence, secondary, 53
intercourse imperative
    assumptions, 4–5
    behavioralism research, 49–50n.5
    biopsychosocial approach,
       100n.36, 100–2
    blaming of women as deficient, 5–7n.30
    consent to sex by women, 5n.17,
       53, 56
    consummation, 56, 66–67
    Freud/psychoanalysis, 64–67
    importance to heterosexual
       relationships, 63–64n.62, 55–64
    loss of male virility treatment, 69n.75
    masturbation as learning tool, 57–58

intercourse imperative (*cont.*)
  men's determination of women's needs, 51–52n.22
  orgasm, Masters/Johnson on, 57–58
  penetration, women's reactions to, 71–72
  penile function, 57
  performance fear, 69–70n.75
  power relationships, 51–55
  pro-male bias, 51–52n.22, 51–55, 62–63, 70–71
  psychological history in research, 66–67
  second wave feminism impacts, 50–51
  sex, women's reactions to, 61–62
  sex as natural function, 64–65
  sex therapy, 58–62, 64–67, 70–71, 92
  sex therapy, structured exercises in, 69n.75, 67–72, 112
  as sexual coercion, 7, 14–15n.62, 51–55, 64
  sexual dysfunctions, 58, 65–67, 70–71
  as social domination tool, 17–18
  spectator role, 69–70n.75
  vagina's biologic readiness, 55–57
  woman's capacity to orgasm as study imperative, 56
  women's enjoyment of by male standards, 5–7n.31, 7–8, 56
  women's sexual motivations, 7
intimate partner violence, 13
Irvine, Janice, 51–52n.22, 57–58

Jackson, Margaret, 4n.13, 16
Johnson, Virginia, 12, 49–50n.5, 51, 64n.62, 91, 92n.14. *See also* intercourse imperative
Jung, Carl, 30

Kahane, Claire, 22
Kaplan, Helen Singer, 12, 14n.61, 49–50, 73–74. *See also* male identification
Katz, Jonathon, 22
Kazin, Alfred, 30
Kinsey, Alfred C., 6, 49, 51, 92n.14
Kleinplatz, Peggy, 6n.25, 16, 113
Koedt, Anne, 33, 51, 55–56
Kroger, William S., 41
Kuhn, Thomas, 120

Lazarus, Arnold A., 93–98, 100
Lazarus, Charles, 144
Leiblum, Sandra R., 49n.5
lesbian couples
  externalization of problem, 153–54
  inequality/power relationships, 148–51
  relationship focus, 151–53
  sex therapy for, 13–14
LoPiccolo, Joseph, 122
Lundberg, Ferdinand, 21n.3, 37

MacKinnon, Catharine, 171
Madden, T. Moore, 2–3
male hypoactive desire disorder, 129
male identification
  agency, 85–86, 87
  equivalency myth, 77n.17, 74–76
  gender domination/victim blaming, 80–81, 83–84
  himpathy, 74, 76, 83
  Kaplan, 73–74
  man's normalcy *vs.* woman's neuroticism, 80, 84, 87
  marriage as bondage, 79–81, 84
  men's sexual sensitivity, 76–79
  rage/yelling/loss of temper, 79–80, 83–84, 143–45
  sex as nutriment, 81–85, 99n.34
  sex as prison, 85–87
  sexual consent, 76
  as therapy paradigm, 73
  third shift, 75–76, 77–78n.17
Malleson, Joan, 88
Manne, Kate, 74
man's prerogative/woman's duty, 15–16, 54–55, 76–79, 80, 87, 111n.7, 115–18n.23. *See also* woman's duty
Marcus, Steven, 22
marriage
  arranged/forced, case study, 85–87
  long-term studies, 145
  loss of feelings, 127–29
  marital rape, 103–4
  sex as precondition, 97–98
  to sexually withholding woman, 14–15n.61
Masters, William, 12, 49–50n.5, 51, 64n.62, 91, 92n.14. *See also* intercourse imperative

masturbation
  Freud's interpretation, 28–31
  historical treatments for, 2–3n.4
  as learning tool, 57–58
  women reaching orgasm via, 6n.25
McCormick, Naomi B., 82n.34
men's sexual sensitivity, 76–79
menstruation taboo, 51–53
#MeToo movement, 174
mindfulness, 158–60
Moi, Toril, 22
Morrison, Toni, 5
Morton, Thomas G., 2–3n.4

normal women standard, 11–12,
  44–46, 167n.2

Oedipal/Electra complex, 25
orgasm
  blaming of women, 113
  clitoris stimulation in, 6, 63–64n.60
  faking, 7, 55, 116–17, 118, 131
  female orgasmic disorder, 112–13,
    138–42, 151
  forbidden/guilty acts, frigidity and, 37
  as indicative of enjoyment, 55
  Masters/Johnson on, 57–58
  masturbation as learning tool, 57–58
  measurement of, 41
  as men's sexual success, 59–60, 69
  orgasmic imperative, 5n.18, 5n.19
  penis-vagina intercourse and,
    5–6n.25, 59–61
  as requirement for women, 5, 7–8n.40
  vaginal, Freud as father of, 33
  vaginal contamination and, 51–53n.22
  woman's attitude, changing, 54–55
Orwell, George, 109
ovariotomy, 2–3

Potts, Annie, 5n.18
power relationships
  assertion of sexual rights, 156–58
  dehumanization, 76–79
  frigidity theory, 32–33n.7, 34–36n.25
  himpathy, 79–80
  intercourse imperative, 51–55
  intersectionality in, 173
  lesbian couples, 148–51

male privilege/dominance, 79–80
man's prerogative/woman's duty, 15–
  16, 54–55, 76–79, 80, 87, 111n.7,
  115–18n.23
19th century views of, 11n.51
sex as ownership of woman, 89–90n.4
social/economic inequality, 7, 13, 15–16
traumatic sexual abuse, 121–24
woman's attitude, changing, 54–55
woman's consent, 53, 56
woman's needs in, 79–81, 83–84
women's socialization/men's privilege/
  power, 169–71
psychiatric disorder, *DSM* definitions of,
  12–13, 163, 167–69

rape/attempted rape, 51–53
relationship focus, 151–53, 161–63, 176
Rich, Adrienne, 116, 131
Richgels, Patricia B., 4n.12
Robinson, Marie N., 32–33, 37, 38,
  43–44, 45–46
Robinson, William Josephus, 42
Rosen, Raymond C., 49n.5
rule of lateral effects, 93–94

Sanger, Margaret, 116
Sedgwick, Eve Kosofsky, 177
self-esteem, dependence upon sex, 7,
  69, 117–18
sensitivity to a man's needs. *See* free
  will of men
sensory experiences
  in sex therapy, 67–72, 91
  in sexual dysfunctions, 112–13
sex therapy
  assertion of sexual rights, 156–58
  autonomy/empowerment in, 155
  change, gentle approach to, 160–61
  distress criterion in diagnosis,
    163–65, 167–68
  equality in diagnosis/resolution, 176
  gender neutrality, 84
  identity power, 16–17
  impaired functioning in
    diagnosis, 168–69
  impotency/Masters/Johnson, 59–60
  incompetent ejaculator/Masters/
    Johnson, 58–59

sex therapy (*cont.*)
   intercourse imperative, 58–62, 64–67, 70–71, 92
   intersectionality in, 173
   mindfulness techniques, 158–60
   miracle question technique, 176–77n.29
   nonorgasmic woman/Masters/Johnson, 60–61
   penile penetration, resistance to, 60–62
   pro-male/anti-female bias in, 7n.31, 8, 12–14, 31, 51–52n.22, 51–55, 76–79, 164–65, 169–70, 171–74n.14
   puzzle-solving model, 120
   reform, 175–77
   relationship focus, 151–53, 161–63, 176
   sensory, 69n.75, 67–72, 91, 112, 127
   sexual desire, teaching, 65
   status quo/patriarchal sexual norm, 16
   strategic ignorance in, 114–18
   structured exercises, Masters/Johnson, 69n.75, 67–72, 112
   women's motivations for seeking, 111n.7, 171
   women's readiness for sex, 82, 99n.34
sexual anorexia, 81–85, 99n.34
sexual coercion
   concepts/definitions of, 115–16n.20, 115–16n.23
   as continuum, 174–75n.24
   damage done by, 147n.44
   intercourse imperative as, 7, 14–15n.62, 51–55, 64
   Masters/Johnson on, 51–52n.22, 51–55
   Nadia/Ivan case study, 129–32, 145
   prevalence, 115–16n.23
   research on, 174
   sex therapy reform, 176
   traumatic sexual abuse, 121–24, 130–32, 143–45
   unacknowledged rape, 171–72n.14
   woman's duty, 147n.44, 143–47
sexual dysfunctions. *See also* sexual coercion
   autonomy/dependence in, 120–21, 128
   consent to sex, 111–12n.8
   consent to sex, enjoyment *vs.*, 115n.18
   dismissal of woman's perspective, 123

   inhibited sexual desire diagnosis, 109–10, 111
   intercourse imperative, 58, 65–67, 70–71
   low sexual desire, stigma removal from, 171
   low sexual desire, therapist's exploration of, 114–15n.18
   pharmacological treatment, 120–21
   as psychiatric disorder, 12–13, 163
   relationship focus, 151–53
   sensory experience, 112–13
   sex therapy, strategic ignorance in, 114–18
   sexual interaction as payment, 115–16n.20
   therapist's inattention to disconfirming evidence, 118–21
   woman's motivation to change, 118–21
sexual energy flow theory, 32–33
sexuality
   pain during copulation, 1–3n.7
   penis-vagina intercourse, universal acceptance of, 4n.14
   power relationships, 19th century views of, 11n.51
   psychiatric discourses on historically, 3–4
   universality of, 4–5, 9, 21
   women's resistance as psychological, 3
Shaw, Jeanne, 16
Shulman, Alix, 64n.60
Sims, J. Marion, 1, 2–3
social scripts, internalization of, 7
societal homophobia, 153–54
Spitzer, Robert L., 109–10, 168–69
Steinbeck, John, 125
Swank, Eric, 77
syphilis, 28–29
systematic desensitization, 92–100, 141–42, 144

Tatchell, Peter, 30
Tiefer, Leonore, 8–9, 16, 167

Umberson, Debra, 115–16n.20, 145

vaginismus, 1–3n.7, 16, 60–62, 99–100, 104n.46, 102–5, 132
value judgments in diagnosis, 168–69
Van de Velde, Theodor, 17, 38, 155

Walker, Rebecca, 71
West, Robin, 147n.44
Wittgenstein, Ludwig, 21
Wolpe, Joseph, 7–8, 12, 49, 92–93, 94n.25, 96–97, 98–99, 100, 144
woman's consent. *See* consent to sex by women
woman's duty
    adaptation of woman to man's desires, 140–42
    background, 137–38
    dismissal of woman's perspective, 138–40
    forced intercourse, 145–47n.44
    husband's behaviors/wife's disinterest, 140–41, 143–47n.44
    ownership of vagina, 142–43
    relational disorder, 138–42
    sexual coercion, 147n.44, 143–47
    systematic desensitization, 141–42, 144

www.ingramcontent.com/pod-product-compliance
Ingram Content Group UK Ltd.
Pitfield, Milton Keynes, MK11 3LW, UK
UKHW022153230426
12049UKWH00003BA/77